DASH DIET COOKBOOK FOR SENIORS

A Comprehensive Guide To Nourishing Recipes, Health Tips, and Meal Plans to Promote Vitality, Well-being, and Longevity"

Linda M. Craig

Copyright © [2024] [Linda M. Craig]

Table of content

Chapter One: Introduction to the DASH Diet

What is the DASH Diet?

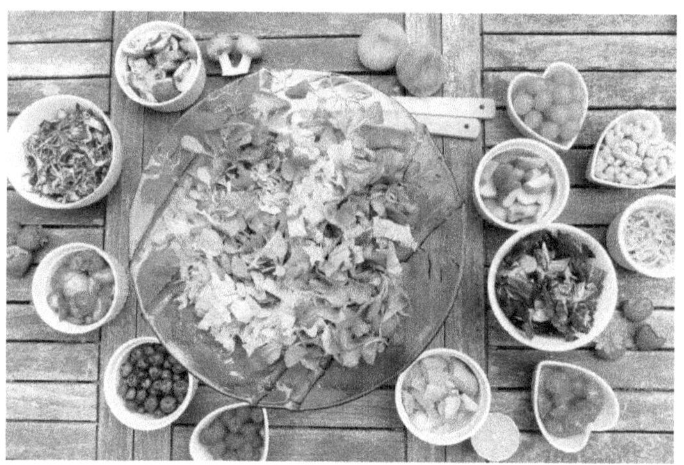

The Dietary Approaches to Stop Hypertension (DASH) diet is a dietary pattern primarily designed to prevent and manage hypertension, or high blood pressure. It emphasizes the consumption of nutrient-rich foods, particularly fruits, vegetables, whole grains, lean proteins, and low-fat dairy products. The DASH diet was developed based on extensive research sponsored by the National Heart, Lung, and Blood Institute (NHLBI), part of the National Institutes of Health (NIH), in the United States.

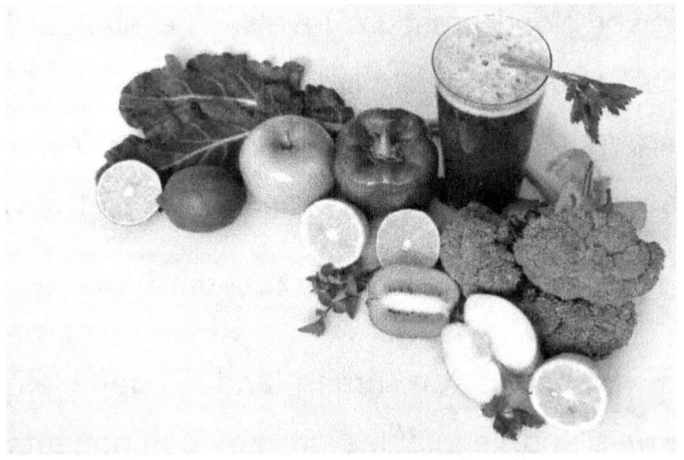

Principles of the DASH Diet:

1. Focus on Nutrient-Rich Foods: The DASH diet encourages the consumption of foods that are rich in essential nutrients such as potassium, magnesium, calcium, and fiber. These include fruits, vegetables, whole

6

grains, nuts, seeds, lean meats, poultry, fish, and low-fat dairy products.

2. Limited Sodium Intake: Sodium, found in salt, is known to contribute to high blood pressure. Therefore, the DASH diet recommends reducing sodium intake to lower blood pressure levels. The standard DASH diet typically limits sodium intake to around 2,300 milligrams per day, but a lower sodium version recommends 1,500 milligrams per day.

3. Emphasis on Fruits and Vegetables: Fruits and vegetables are key components of the DASH diet due to their high content of potassium, magnesium, and fiber, all of which contribute to heart health and blood pressure regulation. The diet encourages a variety of colorful fruits and vegetables to ensure a diverse intake of nutrients.

4. Whole Grains Over Refined Grains: Whole grains, such as brown rice, quinoa, oats, and whole wheat products, are preferred over refined grains like white rice and white bread. Whole grains contain more fiber and nutrients, which can help lower blood pressure and improve overall health.

5. Lean Proteins: Lean proteins, such as poultry, fish, beans, lentils, and tofu, are recommended over red meats and processed meats. These protein sources are lower in saturated fat and cholesterol, making them heart-healthy choices.

6. Moderate Consumption of Dairy: Low-fat or fat-free dairy products, such as milk, yogurt, and cheese, are included in the DASH diet to provide calcium and other essential nutrients. However, portion control

is emphasized to manage calorie and fat intake.

Benefits of the DASH Diet:

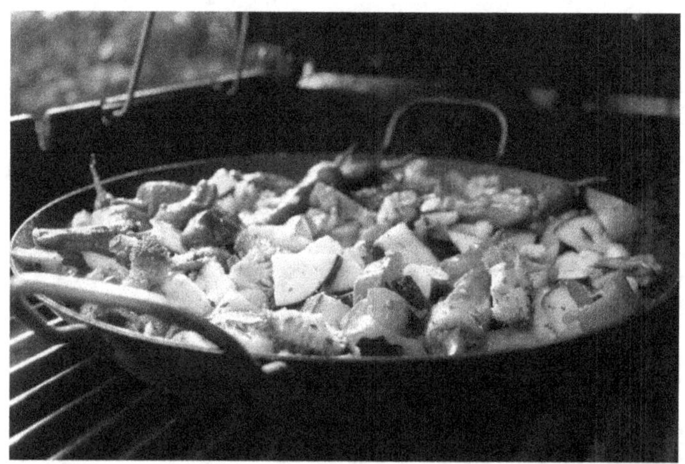

- Blood Pressure Management: Numerous studies have demonstrated the effectiveness of the DASH diet in lowering blood pressure, particularly in individuals with hypertension. Its emphasis on potassium-rich foods and limited sodium intake plays a significant role in reducing blood pressure levels.

- Heart Health: The DASH diet is associated with a reduced risk of cardiovascular disease, including heart attack and stroke. By promoting a balanced and nutrient-rich diet, it helps to improve cholesterol levels, reduce inflammation, and support overall heart health.

- Weight Management: While not specifically designed for weight loss, the DASH diet can aid in weight management due to its focus on whole, nutrient-dense foods. By emphasizing portion control and reducing the consumption of processed and high-calorie foods, individuals may achieve and maintain a healthy weight over time.

- Improved Overall Health: Beyond its impact on blood pressure and heart health, the DASH diet is associated with various other health benefits. These include reduced risk of type 2 diabetes, improved insulin sensitivity, better digestion due to increased fiber intake, and enhanced immune function.

Benefits of the DASH Diet for Seniors

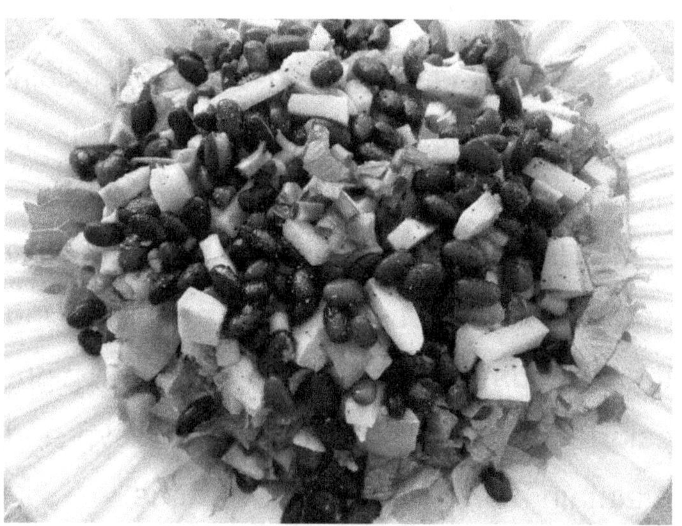

As individuals age, maintaining optimal health becomes increasingly important. The Dietary Approaches to Stop Hypertension (DASH) diet offers numerous benefits for seniors, helping to address age-related health concerns and improve overall well-being. Below is a detailed exploration of the benefits of the DASH diet specifically tailored to seniors:

1. Blood Pressure Management:
   - Hypertension, or high blood pressure, is common among seniors and can increase the risk of cardiovascular disease and other health complications. The DASH diet's emphasis on potassium-rich foods, such as fruits and vegetables, and its restriction of sodium intake can effectively lower blood pressure levels in seniors.
   - Research has consistently shown that adherence to the DASH diet can lead to significant reductions in both systolic and diastolic blood pressure, reducing the risk of stroke, heart attack, and other cardiovascular events in seniors.

2. Heart Health:

- Seniors are particularly vulnerable to heart-related conditions, making heart health a top priority. The DASH diet promotes heart health by encouraging the consumption of nutrient-rich foods that support cardiovascular function, such as whole grains, lean proteins, and unsaturated fats.

- By incorporating heart-healthy foods and limiting saturated and trans fats, the DASH diet can help seniors maintain healthy cholesterol levels, reduce inflammation, and improve overall cardiac function, lowering the risk of heart disease and related complications.

3. Weight Management:

- Many seniors struggle with weight management due to factors such as decreased metabolism, reduced physical activity, and changes in appetite. The DASH diet provides a balanced and sustainable approach to weight management, emphasizing whole, nutrient-dense foods while limiting processed and high-calorie options.

- By promoting portion control, increasing fiber intake, and focusing on foods that promote satiety, the DASH diet can help seniors achieve and maintain a healthy weight. This is essential for reducing the risk of obesity-related conditions such as type 2 diabetes, joint pain, and mobility issues.

4. Nutrient-Rich Diet:

- As individuals age, nutrient absorption and utilization may decline, increasing the risk of nutrient deficiencies. The DASH diet prioritizes nutrient-rich foods, including fruits, vegetables, whole grains, lean proteins, and low-fat dairy products, to ensure seniors receive essential vitamins, minerals, and antioxidants.

   - By consuming a diverse array of nutrient-dense foods, seniors can support immune function, maintain bone health, preserve cognitive function, and enhance overall vitality, promoting a higher quality of life as they age.

5. Reduced Risk of Chronic Diseases:

   - Seniors are at a higher risk of developing chronic diseases such as type 2 diabetes, osteoporosis, and certain cancers. The DASH diet, with its focus on whole, unprocessed foods and balanced nutrition, can help reduce the risk of these conditions and their associated complications.

   - Studies have shown that adherence to the DASH diet is associated with a lower incidence of type 2 diabetes, improved insulin sensitivity, and better management of blood sugar levels in seniors. Additionally, the diet's emphasis on calcium-rich foods can support bone health and reduce the risk of osteoporosis.

6. Enhanced Quality of Life:

- Beyond its physical health benefits, the DASH diet can also enhance seniors' overall quality of life by promoting mental well-being, cognitive function, and independence. A diet rich in fruits, vegetables, and whole grains has been linked to improved mood, cognitive performance, and longevity.

- By providing sustained energy levels, supporting healthy digestion, and reducing inflammation, the DASH diet enables seniors to stay active, engaged, and independent for longer, allowing them to enjoy a fulfilling and vibrant lifestyle as they age.

Getting Started with the DASH Diet

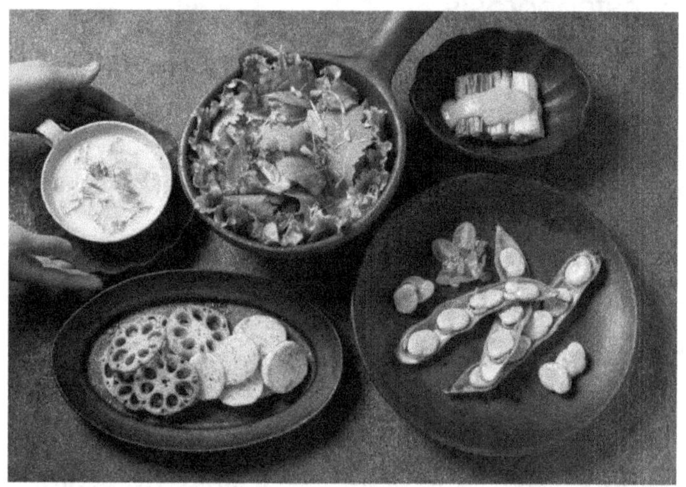

Embarking on the Dietary Approaches to Stop Hypertension (DASH) diet can be a transformative journey toward better health and well-being. Whether you're looking to manage hypertension, improve heart health, or simply adopt a more nutritious eating pattern, getting started with the DASH diet involves understanding its principles, setting realistic goals, and making gradual changes to your diet and lifestyle. Below is a detailed overview of how to begin your journey with the DASH diet:

1. Understand the Principles of the DASH Diet:

- The DASH diet emphasizes the consumption of nutrient-rich foods, such as fruits, vegetables, whole grains, lean proteins, and low-fat dairy products.

- It limits the intake of sodium, saturated fats, refined grains, and sugary beverages, all of which can contribute to high blood pressure and other health issues.

- The diet encourages portion control, balanced meals, and mindful eating habits to promote overall health and well-being.

2. Assess Your Current Diet and Lifestyle:

- Before starting the DASH diet, take stock of your current eating habits and lifestyle choices. Keep a food diary for a few days to track your intake of fruits, vegetables, whole grains, and other key food groups, as well as your sodium consumption.

- Consider factors such as physical activity level, stress management, sleep quality, and hydration habits, as these can all impact your overall health and the effectiveness of the DASH diet.

3. Set Realistic Goals:

- Determine what you hope to achieve by adopting the DASH diet. Whether it's lowering your blood pressure, improving your cholesterol levels, losing weight, or simply feeling more energized and vibrant, setting clear and achievable goals will help you stay motivated and focused.

- Start with small, attainable goals and gradually increase the intensity and duration as you progress. Celebrate your successes along the way and be patient with yourself as you navigate the transition to a healthier lifestyle.

4. Educate Yourself About DASH-Friendly Foods:

- Familiarize yourself with the types of foods that are encouraged and discouraged on the DASH diet. Stock your kitchen with plenty of fruits, vegetables, whole grains, lean proteins, and low-fat dairy products.

- Experiment with new recipes and cooking techniques to make meals more flavorful and enjoyable. Explore different herbs, spices, and seasonings to enhance the natural flavors of your dishes without relying on excess salt or unhealthy fats.

5. Plan Your Meals and Snacks:

- Planning is key to success on the DASH diet. Take time each week to create a meal plan that includes a variety of DASH-friendly foods and recipes.

- Aim for balanced meals that incorporate a mix of carbohydrates, protein, and healthy fats. Include plenty of fruits and vegetables at each meal, and opt for whole grains over refined grains whenever possible.

- Prepare healthy snacks to have on hand for times when hunger strikes between meals. Choose nutrient-dense options such as fresh fruit, raw vegetables with hummus, Greek yogurt, nuts, or whole grain crackers with cheese.

6. Monitor Your Progress and Adjust as Needed:

- Keep track of your progress on the DASH diet by monitoring your blood pressure, weight, and other relevant health markers. Use a journal or app to record your food intake, physical activity, and any symptoms or changes you notice.

- Be flexible and willing to adjust your approach as needed based on your individual preferences, goals, and feedback from your healthcare provider. Remember that the DASH diet is not a one-size-fits-all approach, and what works for one person may need to be modified for another.

7. Seek Support and Accountability:

- Enlist the support of friends, family members, or a healthcare professional to help you stay accountable and motivated on your DASH diet journey. Share your goals and challenges with others who can offer encouragement, advice, and practical support.

- Consider joining a DASH diet support group or online community where you can connect with like-minded individuals, share experiences, and exchange ideas for success.

Getting started with the DASH diet is a proactive step toward improving your health and well-being. By understanding the principles of the diet, setting realistic goals, educating yourself about DASH-friendly foods, planning your meals and snacks, monitoring your progress, and seeking support and accountability, you can lay the foundation for long-term success and sustainable lifestyle changes. Remember that small, consistent changes over time can lead to significant improvements in your health and quality of life.

Chapter Two: DASH Diet Basics for Seniors

Understanding Macronutrients and Micronutrients

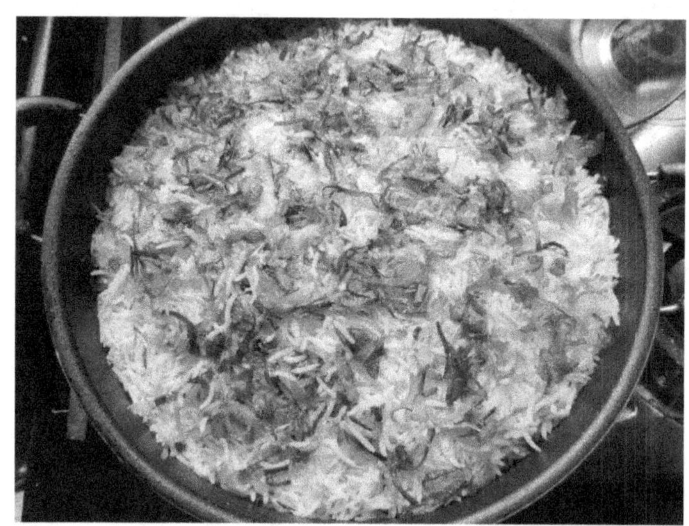

Nutrients are essential substances that our bodies require for growth, development, and overall health. They can be broadly categorized into two main groups: macronutrients and micronutrients.

Understanding the roles, sources, and importance of both macronutrients and micronutrients is crucial for maintaining a balanced and nutritious diet. Below is a detailed exploration of these two categories of nutrients:

Macronutrients:

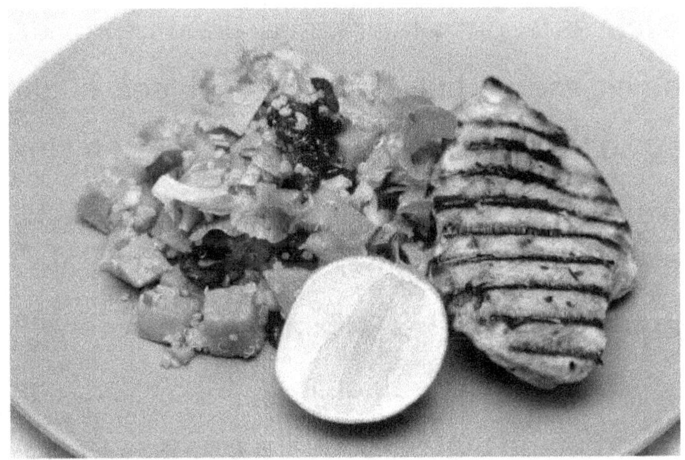

Macronutrients are nutrients that provide energy (calories) and are needed by the body in relatively large amounts. There are three main macronutrients:

1. Carbohydrates:

- Carbohydrates are the body's primary source of energy. They are found in a wide variety of foods, including grains, fruits, vegetables, legumes, and dairy products.

- Carbohydrates can be categorized as simple or complex, depending on their chemical structure. Simple carbohydrates, such as sugar and refined grains, provide quick energy but may lead to blood sugar spikes and crashes. Complex carbohydrates, found in whole grains, fruits, and vegetables, provide sustained energy and are rich in fiber, vitamins, and minerals.

- The Dietary Guidelines for Americans recommend that carbohydrates make up 45-65% of total daily calories, with an emphasis on choosing whole, unprocessed sources whenever possible.

2. Proteins:

- Proteins are essential for building and repairing tissues, producing enzymes and hormones, and supporting immune function. They are composed of amino acids, which are often referred to as the "building blocks" of protein.

- Dietary sources of protein include meat, poultry, fish, eggs, dairy products, legumes, nuts, and seeds. Animal-based proteins tend to be complete, meaning they contain all essential amino acids, while plant-based proteins may be incomplete and need to be combined to ensure adequate intake of all amino acids.

- The recommended dietary allowance (RDA) for protein varies based on factors such as age, sex, weight, and activity level, but generally ranges from 0.8 to 1.0 grams of protein per kilogram of body weight per day.

3. Fats:

- Fats are a concentrated source of energy and are essential for various bodily functions, including hormone production, cell membrane integrity, and nutrient absorption.

- There are different types of fats, including saturated fats, unsaturated fats (monounsaturated and polyunsaturated), and trans fats. Saturated and trans fats are considered less healthy and are found in foods such as butter, cheese, red meat, and processed snacks. Unsaturated fats, on the other hand, are found in foods such as nuts, seeds, avocados, and fatty fish and are associated with numerous health benefits, including heart health.

- The Dietary Guidelines for Americans recommend that fats make up 20-35% of total daily calories, with an emphasis on choosing unsaturated fats and limiting saturated and trans fats.

Micronutrients:

Micronutrients are nutrients that are required by the body in smaller amounts but are essential for various physiological processes. They include vitamins and minerals, which play crucial roles in metabolism, immune function, bone health, and many other functions. Here's a closer look at micronutrients:

1. Vitamins:

   - Vitamins are organic compounds that are essential for normal growth, development, and overall health. There are 13 essential vitamins, each with its own unique functions and dietary sources.

   - Vitamins can be classified as water-soluble (such as vitamin C and the B vitamins) or fat-soluble (such as vitamins A, D, E, and K), depending on their solubility in water or fat.

   - Water-soluble vitamins are not stored in the body and need to be consumed regularly through the diet, while fat-soluble vitamins can be stored in the body's fat tissues and liver for longer periods.

2. Minerals:

   - Minerals are inorganic elements that are essential for various bodily functions, including bone health, nerve function, fluid balance, and muscle contraction.
   - There are two main categories of minerals: macrominerals, which are needed in larger amounts (e.g., calcium, magnesium, potassium, sodium), and trace minerals, which are required in smaller amounts (e.g., iron, zinc, copper, selenium).

- Minerals are found in a wide variety of foods, including fruits, vegetables, whole grains, dairy products, meat, poultry, fish, nuts, and seeds. Some minerals, such as calcium and iron, may be more challenging to obtain in adequate amounts through diet alone, and supplementation may be necessary for certain individuals.

Importance of Balance:
Both macronutrients and micronutrients play essential roles in maintaining overall health and well-being. A balanced diet that provides adequate amounts of carbohydrates, proteins, fats, vitamins, and minerals is essential for supporting growth, energy production, immune function, and disease prevention.

Guidelines for Senior-Specific Nutrition on the DASH Diet

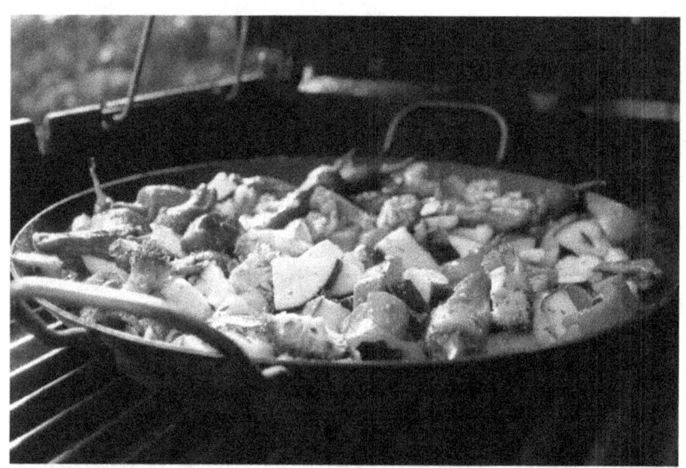

As individuals age, their nutritional needs and dietary considerations may change, making it important to adapt dietary patterns accordingly. The Dietary Approaches to Stop Hypertension (DASH) diet offers seniors a flexible and effective approach to improving their health and well-being while addressing age-related concerns. Below are detailed guidelines for senior-specific nutrition on the DASH diet:

1. Emphasize Nutrient-Dense Foods:

- Seniors should prioritize nutrient-dense foods to meet their changing nutritional needs. Focus on incorporating plenty of fruits, vegetables, whole grains, lean proteins, and low-fat dairy products into meals and snacks.

- These foods provide essential vitamins, minerals, antioxidants, and fiber, which are important for maintaining overall health, supporting immune function, and preventing chronic diseases commonly associated with aging.

2. Adjust Caloric Intake as Needed:

- As metabolism tends to slow down with age, seniors may need to adjust their caloric intake to prevent weight gain and maintain a healthy weight. Pay attention to portion sizes and energy needs, being mindful of changes in activity level and metabolism.

- Choose nutrient-dense, lower-calorie foods to fill up on, such as fruits, vegetables, and lean proteins, while limiting higher-calorie foods and beverages that provide little nutritional value.

3. Monitor Sodium Intake:

- Seniors are often more susceptible to the negative effects of high sodium intake, including hypertension, fluid retention, and kidney problems. Therefore, it's essential to monitor sodium intake and adhere to the recommended limits outlined in the DASH diet.

- Opt for fresh or minimally processed foods and season meals with herbs, spices, and citrus juices instead of salt. Limit the consumption of processed and packaged foods, which tend to be high in sodium.

4. Prioritize Heart-Healthy Fats:

- Healthy fats play a crucial role in supporting heart health and cognitive function in seniors. Choose sources of unsaturated fats, such as olive oil, avocado, nuts, seeds, and fatty fish, which provide omega-3 fatty acids and other beneficial nutrients.

- Limit saturated and trans fats found in fried foods, processed snacks, red meat, and full-fat dairy products, as these fats can contribute to heart disease and other health issues.

5. Focus on Calcium and Vitamin D:

- Calcium and vitamin D are essential for maintaining bone health and preventing osteoporosis, a common concern for seniors. Ensure an adequate intake of calcium-rich foods, such as low-fat dairy products, leafy greens, fortified cereals, and canned fish with bones.

 - Additionally, aim to get enough vitamin D through sunlight exposure and dietary sources like fatty fish, fortified dairy products, and vitamin D supplements if necessary, as vitamin D helps the body absorb calcium.

6. Stay Hydrated:

 - Dehydration can be a concern for seniors, especially as the sense of thirst may decrease with age. Make a conscious effort to stay hydrated by drinking plenty of fluids throughout the day, including water, herbal teas, and low-sugar beverages.

 - Monitor fluid intake, particularly in hot weather or during physical activity, and be aware of signs of dehydration, such as dry mouth, dark urine, and dizziness. Aim to consume fluids with meals and snacks to ensure adequate hydration.

7. Consider Individual Needs and Preferences:

- Seniors may have unique dietary preferences, restrictions, or health conditions that need to be taken into account when following the DASH diet. Work with a healthcare provider or registered dietitian to tailor a nutrition plan that meets individual needs and goals.

- Take into consideration factors such as chewing and swallowing difficulties, medication interactions, food allergies or intolerances, and cultural or religious dietary practices when planning meals and snacks.

8. Promote Social and Emotional Well-Being:

- Nutrition is not just about physical health but also plays a significant role in social and emotional well-being for seniors. Encourage socialization and enjoyment of meals by dining with family or friends, participating in community events, and exploring new recipes and cuisines.

- Maintain a positive attitude toward food and eating, and approach mealtime as an opportunity to nourish the body and soul. Celebrate food as a source of pleasure, connection, and vitality, and savor the flavors and experiences that come with it.

Following these guidelines for senior-specific nutrition on the DASH diet can help optimize health, well-being, and quality of life for older adults. By prioritizing nutrient-dense foods, monitoring sodium intake, choosing heart-healthy fats, prioritizing bone health, staying hydrated, considering individual needs and preferences, and promoting social and emotional well-being, seniors can enjoy the benefits of the DASH diet while maintaining independence and vitality as they age. Working with healthcare providers and registered dietitians can provide additional support and guidance tailored to individual needs and goals.

Meal Planning and Preparation Tips for Seniors

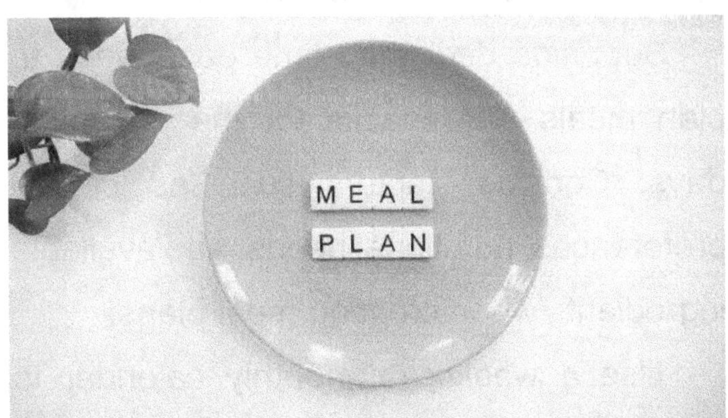

Meal planning and preparation are essential components of successfully adopting and maintaining a healthy dietary pattern like the Dietary Approaches to Stop Hypertension (DASH) diet, especially for seniors. By incorporating practical strategies and tips into their meal planning and preparation routines, seniors can make nutritious eating more accessible, enjoyable, and sustainable. Below are detailed guidelines for meal planning and preparation tailored to seniors following the DASH diet:

1. Plan Meals Ahead of Time:

- Set aside dedicated time each week to plan meals and snacks for the upcoming days. Consider factors such as dietary preferences, nutritional needs, and available ingredients when creating meal plans.

- Use a weekly or monthly calendar to outline meals and snacks for each day, taking into account any social events, appointments, or activities that may impact mealtime availability.

2. Incorporate Variety and Balance:

- Aim for a diverse array of foods from all food groups to ensure adequate nutrient intake and prevent dietary monotony. Include a mix of fruits, vegetables, whole grains, lean proteins, and low-fat dairy products in meals and snacks.

- Experiment with different recipes, cooking methods, and cuisines to keep meals interesting and enjoyable. Use herbs, spices, and seasonings to enhance flavors without relying on excess salt or unhealthy fats.

3. Opt for Batch Cooking and Freezing:

- Simplify meal preparation by batch cooking larger quantities of staple foods and freezing individual portions for later use.

Cook grains, beans, soups, stews, and casseroles in large batches and portion them out into freezer-safe containers for convenient meals and snacks.

- Label and date frozen meals for easy identification and rotation, and consider investing in portion-sized freezer bags or containers to minimize waste and ensure proper portion control.

4. Choose Convenient and Time-Saving Ingredients:

- Select convenience foods and ingredients that require minimal preparation and cooking time, such as pre-cut fruits and vegetables, canned beans, pre-cooked grains, frozen vegetables, and rotisserie chicken.

- Stock your pantry with healthy staples like whole grain pasta, brown rice, quinoa, canned tomatoes, low-sodium broth, and canned tuna or salmon to create quick and nutritious meals on busy days.

5. Use Kitchen Gadgets and Appliances:

- Take advantage of kitchen gadgets and appliances to streamline meal preparation and cooking processes. Invest in a slow cooker, pressure cooker, blender, food processor, or microwave oven to make cooking easier and more efficient.

- Experiment with different cooking methods, such as steaming, roasting, grilling, or sautéing, to enhance flavors and textures while preserving nutrients in foods.

6. Practice Portion Control and Mindful Eating:

- Be mindful of portion sizes and practice portion control to avoid overeating and promote satiety. Use smaller plates, bowls, and utensils to visually cue appropriate portion sizes and prevent excessive calorie intake.

- Eat slowly, savoring each bite, and pay attention to hunger and fullness cues to prevent mindless eating and promote better digestion. Aim to stop eating when you feel comfortably satisfied, rather than overly full.

7. Involve Others and Share Meals:

- Engage family members, friends, or caregivers in meal planning and preparation activities to foster social connection and teamwork. Share cooking responsibilities, exchange recipe ideas, and enjoy meals together as a way to bond and support each other's health goals.

- Consider participating in community meal programs, meal delivery services, or potluck gatherings to access nutritious meals and connect with peers in a supportive environment.

8. Adapt Recipes to Dietary Needs and Preferences:

- Modify recipes to accommodate individual dietary needs, preferences, and restrictions, such as food allergies, intolerances, or medical conditions. Substitute ingredients as needed and adjust seasonings and flavors to suit personal taste preferences.

- Seek out DASH-friendly recipes specifically designed for seniors or individuals with specific dietary considerations, and don't hesitate to experiment with ingredient substitutions and modifications to make recipes more accessible and enjoyable.

By including these meal planning and preparation tips into their daily routines, seniors can enhance their adherence to the

DASH diet while promoting health, convenience, and enjoyment. By planning ahead, incorporating variety and balance, using time-saving ingredients and kitchen gadgets, practicing portion control and mindful eating, involving others and sharing meals, and adapting recipes to individual needs and preferences, seniors can make nutritious eating a sustainable and fulfilling part of their lives. Working with a healthcare provider or registered dietitian can provide additional support and guidance tailored to individual needs and goals.

Chapter Three: Delicious DASH Diet Recipes for Seniors

Breakfast Recipes

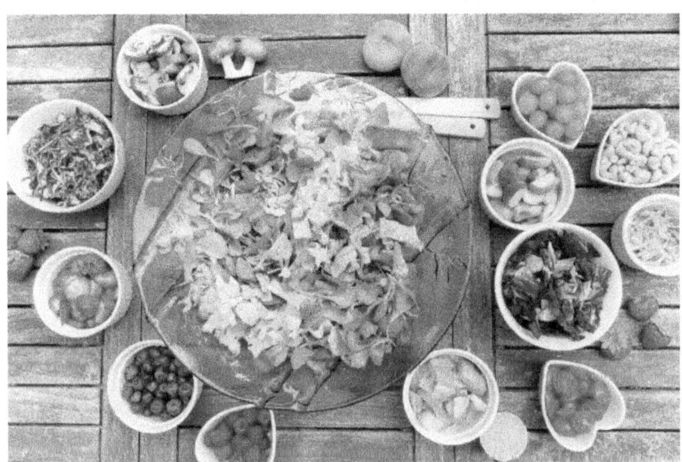

Breakfast is often considered the most important meal of the day, providing essential nutrients and energy to kickstart your morning and set the tone for the day ahead. Incorporating DASH-friendly breakfast recipes into your morning routine can help you meet your nutritional goals while enjoying delicious and satisfying meals. Below are detailed recipes for nutritious breakfast options tailored to the DASH diet:

1. Greek Yogurt Parfait:

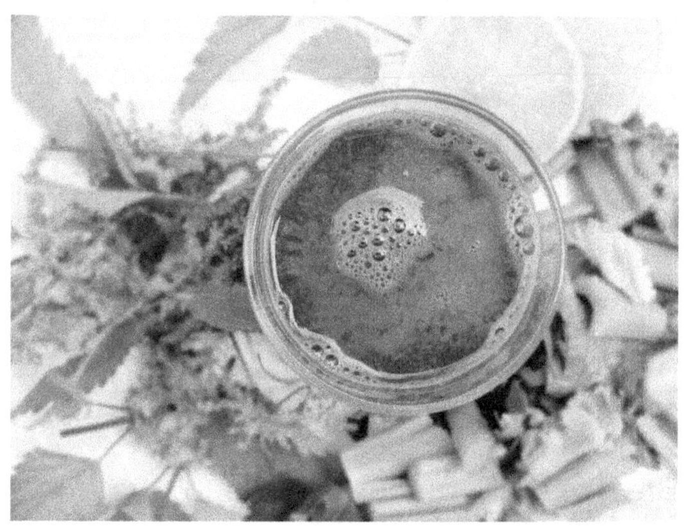

   - Ingredients:

     - 1/2 cup plain Greek yogurt

     - 1/4 cup fresh berries (such as strawberries, blueberries, or raspberries)

     - 1 tablespoon honey or maple syrup (optional)

- 2 tablespoons granola or crushed nuts

- Instructions:

1. In a serving glass or bowl, layer Greek yogurt, fresh berries, and honey or maple syrup (if using).

2. Top with granola or crushed nuts for added crunch and texture.

3. Enjoy immediately as a refreshing and protein-packed breakfast option.

2. Veggie Omelette:

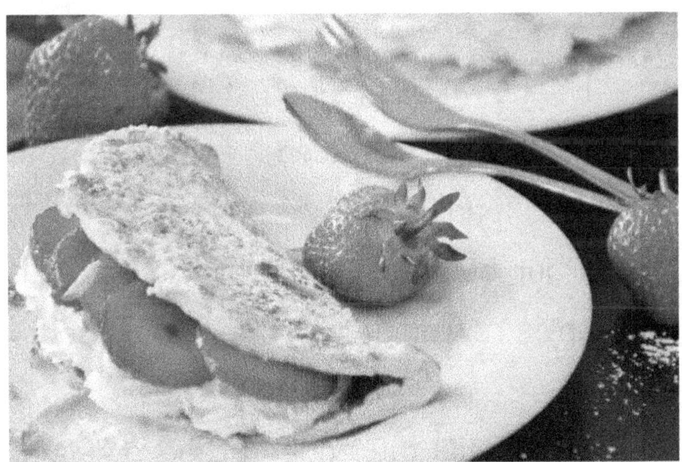

- Ingredients:

  - 2 large eggs

  - 1/4 cup diced bell peppers

  - 1/4 cup diced tomatoes

  - 1/4 cup chopped spinach

  - 1 tablespoon chopped onion

  - Salt and pepper to taste

  - 1 teaspoon olive oil

- Instructions:

1. In a small bowl, beat the eggs until well combined. Season with salt and pepper to taste.

2. Heat olive oil in a non-stick skillet over medium heat. Add diced vegetables and sauté until tender.

3. Pour beaten eggs over the sautéed vegetables, swirling the skillet to distribute evenly.

4. Cook until the edges of the omelette are set and the center is slightly runny. Use a spatula to fold the omelette in half.

5. Cook for an additional minute or until the eggs are fully cooked through.

6. Serve hot with a side of whole grain toast or fresh fruit for a hearty and nutritious breakfast.

3. Whole Grain Pancakes:

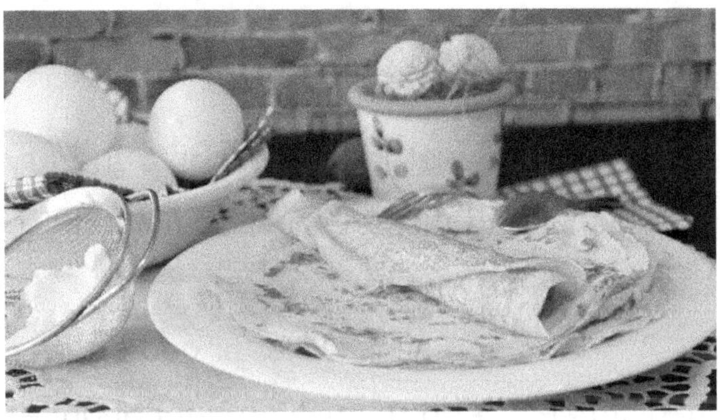

- Ingredients:

- 1 cup whole wheat flour

- 1 tablespoon baking powder

- 1 tablespoon honey or maple syrup

- 1 cup low-fat milk or unsweetened almond milk

- 1 large egg

- 1 tablespoon unsalted butter or olive oil

- Optional toppings: fresh fruit, Greek yogurt, nuts, or pure maple syrup

- Instructions:

1. In a large mixing bowl, whisk together whole wheat flour and baking powder.

2. In a separate bowl, whisk together honey or maple syrup, milk, and egg until well combined.

3. Pour the wet ingredients into the dry ingredients and mix until just combined. Be careful not to overmix.

4. Heat a non-stick skillet or griddle over medium heat. Add a small amount of butter or olive oil to coat the surface.

5. Pour 1/4 cup of pancake batter onto the skillet and cook until bubbles form on the surface. Flip the pancake and cook until golden brown on both sides.

6. Repeat with the remaining batter, adding more butter or oil to the skillet as needed.

7. Serve warm with your choice of toppings for a wholesome and satisfying breakfast option.

4. Overnight Oats:

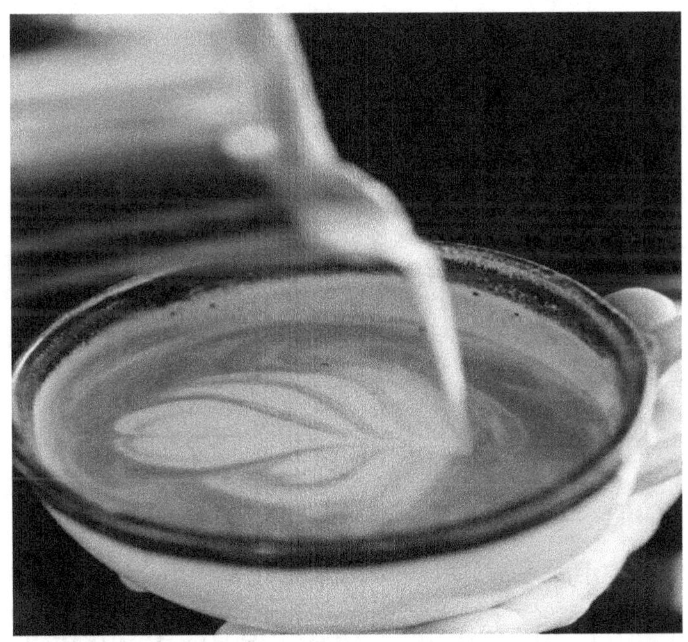

- Ingredients:

  - 1/2 cup rolled oats

  - 1/2 cup low-fat milk or unsweetened almond milk

  - 1/4 cup plain Greek yogurt

  - 1 tablespoon chia seeds

  - 1 tablespoon honey or maple syrup

  - Optional add-ins: fresh fruit, nuts, seeds, or spices (such as cinnamon or nutmeg)

- Instructions:

  1. In a mason jar or airtight container, combine rolled oats, milk, Greek yogurt, chia seeds, and honey or maple syrup.

  2. Stir until well combined, then cover and refrigerate overnight or for at least 4 hours to allow the oats to soften and absorb the liquid.

  3. In the morning, give the overnight oats a stir and adjust the consistency with additional milk if desired.

4. Top with your favorite add-ins, such as fresh fruit, nuts, seeds, or spices, for added flavor and texture.

5. Enjoy cold straight from the fridge or heat in the microwave for a warm and comforting breakfast option.

5. Spinach and Feta Breakfast Wrap:

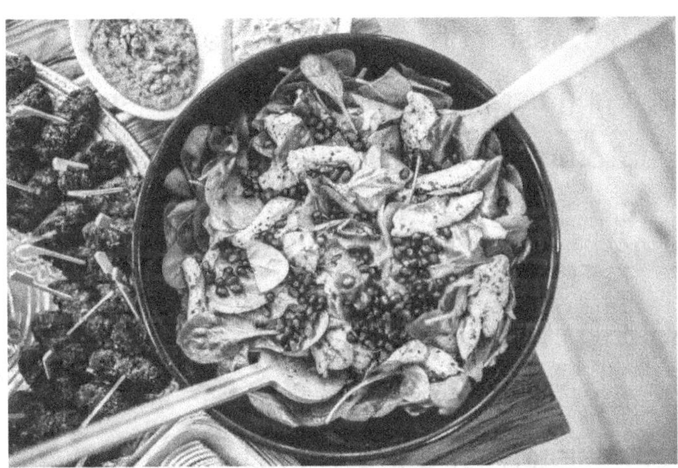

- Ingredients:

    - 1 whole grain tortilla

    - 2 large eggs, scrambled

    - 1/4 cup chopped spinach

    - 2 tablespoons crumbled feta cheese

- Salt and pepper to taste

- Instructions:

1. Heat a whole grain tortilla in a dry skillet over medium heat until warm and slightly toasted.

2. In a separate skillet, scramble the eggs until cooked through. Season with salt and pepper to taste.

3. Assemble the breakfast wrap by layering scrambled eggs, chopped spinach, and crumbled feta cheese on the warmed tortilla.

4. Roll up the tortilla to enclose the filling, folding in the sides as you go.

5. Slice the wrap in half and serve immediately for a protein-rich and satisfying breakfast on the go.

Adding these delicious and nutritious breakfast recipes into your morning routine can help you start your day off on the right foot while following the DASH diet. By choosing whole, nutrient-dense ingredients and incorporating a variety of flavors and textures, you can enjoy satisfying meals that support your health and well-being. Experiment with different recipes and adapt them to suit your taste preferences and dietary needs for a truly enjoyable breakfast experience.

Lunch Recipes

Lunch is an important opportunity to refuel your body and provide it with the nutrients it needs to sustain energy levels and promote overall health and well-being. Incorporating DASH-friendly lunch recipes into your midday meals can help you maintain a balanced diet while enjoying delicious and satisfying dishes. Below are detailed recipes for nutritious lunch options tailored to the DASH diet:

1. Quinoa Salad with Chickpeas and Vegetables:

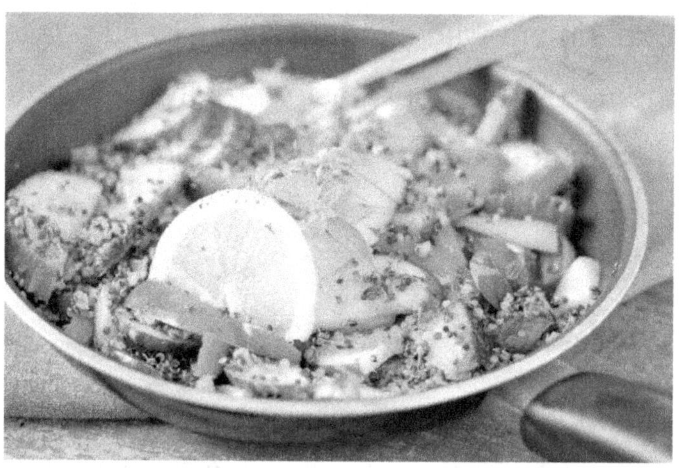

- Ingredients:

  - 1 cup cooked quinoa

  - 1/2 cup cooked chickpeas (canned, drained, and rinsed)

  - 1 cup chopped mixed vegetables (such as bell peppers, cucumbers, cherry tomatoes, and red onion)

- 2 tablespoons chopped fresh herbs (such as parsley, cilantro, or basil)

- 2 tablespoons extra-virgin olive oil

- 1 tablespoon lemon juice

- Salt and pepper to taste

- Instructions:

1. In a large mixing bowl, combine cooked quinoa, chickpeas, chopped vegetables, and fresh herbs.

2. In a small bowl, whisk together olive oil, lemon juice, salt, and pepper to make the dressing.

3. Pour the dressing over the quinoa salad and toss until well coated.

4. Serve chilled or at room temperature as a hearty and nutritious lunch option.

2. Turkey and Avocado Wrap:

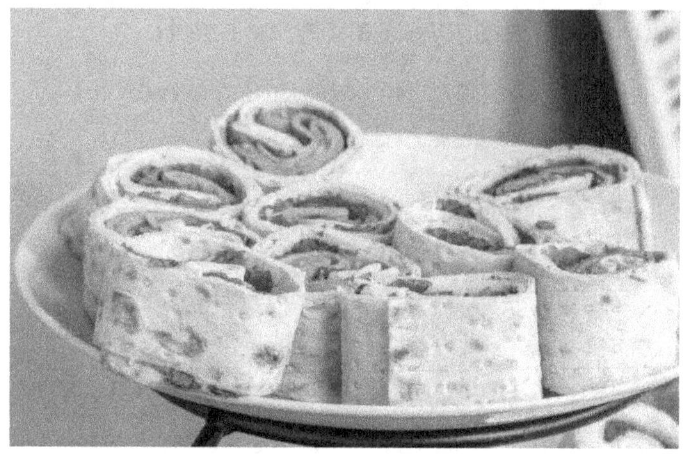

- Ingredients:

- 1 whole grain tortilla

- 2 slices roasted turkey breast

- 1/4 avocado, sliced

- 1/4 cup shredded lettuce

- 2 slices tomato

- 1 tablespoon hummus or Greek yogurt spread

- Instructions:

1. Lay the whole grain tortilla flat on a clean surface.

2. Spread hummus or Greek yogurt evenly over the tortilla.

3. Layer roasted turkey breast, avocado slices, shredded lettuce, and tomato slices on top of the spread.

4. Roll up the tortilla to enclose the filling, folding in the sides as you go.

5. Slice the wrap in half and secure with toothpicks if necessary.

6. Serve immediately as a protein-rich and satisfying lunch option.

3. Lentil and Vegetable Soup:

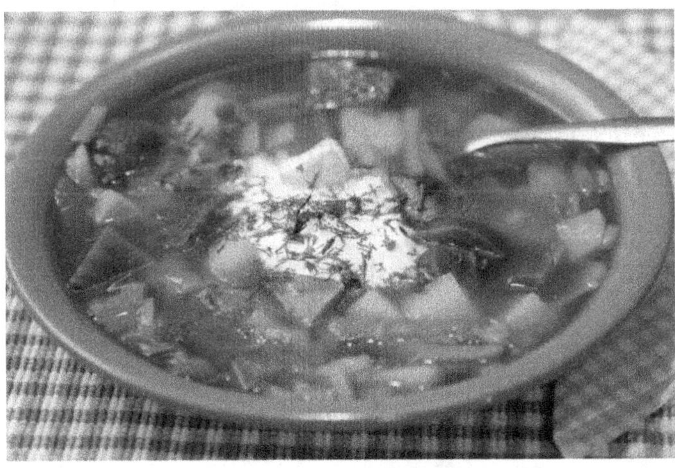

- Ingredients:

    - 1 tablespoon olive oil

    - 1/2 cup chopped onion

    - 1/2 cup chopped carrots

    - 1/2 cup chopped celery

    - 2 cloves garlic, minced

    - 1 cup dried green or brown lentils, rinsed and drained

    - 4 cups low-sodium vegetable or chicken broth

    - 1 bay leaf

    - 1 teaspoon dried thyme

    - Salt and pepper to taste

    - 2 cups chopped kale or spinach

- Instructions:

    1. Heat olive oil in a large pot over medium heat. Add chopped onion, carrots, and celery, and sauté until softened.

    2. Add minced garlic and cook for an additional minute until fragrant.

3. Stir in dried lentils, vegetable or chicken broth, bay leaf, dried thyme, salt, and pepper.

4. Bring the soup to a boil, then reduce heat to low and simmer for 20-25 minutes, or until lentils are tender.

5. Add chopped kale or spinach to the soup during the last 5 minutes of cooking, stirring until wilted.

6. Remove the bay leaf and adjust seasoning as needed before serving.

7. Ladle the soup into bowls and enjoy hot as a comforting and nutritious lunch option.

4. Grilled Chicken Salad with Balsamic Vinaigrette:

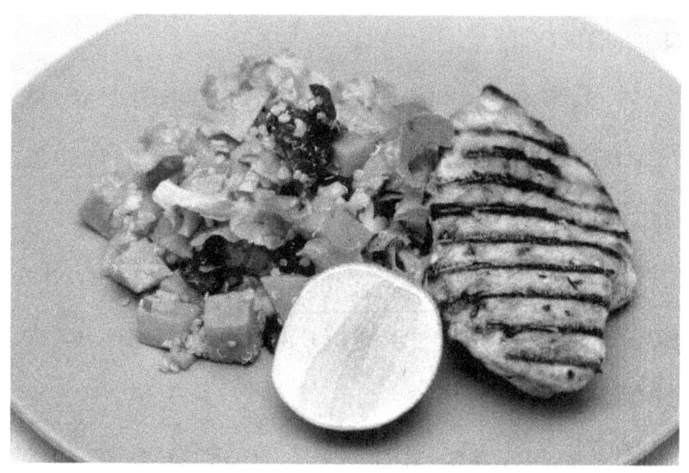

- Ingredients:

    - 4 ounces grilled chicken breast, sliced

    - 2 cups mixed salad greens

    - 1/2 cup cherry tomatoes, halved

    - 1/4 cup sliced cucumber

    - 1/4 cup sliced bell peppers

    - 2 tablespoons crumbled feta cheese

    - 1 tablespoon chopped walnuts or almonds

    - 2 tablespoons balsamic vinaigrette dressing

- Instructions:

1. Arrange mixed salad greens on a serving plate or bowl.

2. Top with grilled chicken breast slices, cherry tomatoes, sliced cucumber, sliced bell peppers, crumbled feta cheese, and chopped nuts.

3. Drizzle balsamic vinaigrette dressing over the salad.

4. Toss gently to combine, ensuring all ingredients are evenly coated with dressing.

5. Serve immediately as a protein-packed and satisfying lunch option.

5. Mediterranean Veggie Wrap:

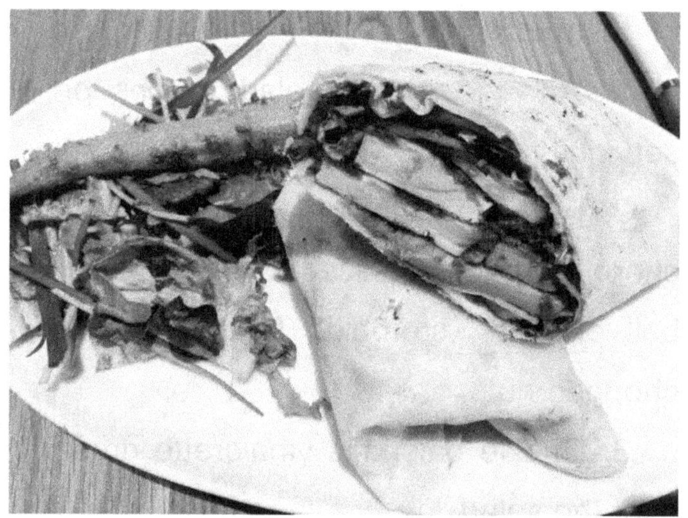

- Ingredients:

  - 1 whole grain tortilla

  - 2 tablespoons hummus

  - 1/4 cup diced cucumber

  - 1/4 cup diced tomatoes

  - 2 tablespoons sliced black olives

  - 2 tablespoons crumbled feta cheese

  - 1 tablespoon chopped fresh parsley or basil

- Instructions:

  1. Spread hummus evenly over the whole grain tortilla.

2. Layer diced cucumber, diced tomatoes, sliced black olives, crumbled feta cheese, and chopped fresh herbs on top of the hummus.

3. Roll up the tortilla to enclose the filling, folding in the sides as you go.

4. Slice the wrap in half and serve immediately for a flavorful and nutrient-rich lunch option.

Including these delicious and nutritious lunch recipes into your meal rotation can help you maintain a balanced and satisfying diet while following the DASH guidelines. By choosing whole, nutrient-dense ingredients and incorporating a variety of flavors and textures, you can enjoy nourishing meals that support your health and well-being. Experiment with different recipes and adapt them to suit your taste preferences and dietary needs for a truly enjoyable lunchtime experience.

Dinner Recipes

Dinner is an opportunity to unwind and nourish your body with a balanced and nutritious meal, especially when following the Dietary Approaches to Stop Hypertension (DASH) diet. Incorporating DASH-friendly dinner recipes into your evening routine can help you maintain optimal health while enjoying delicious and satisfying dishes. Below are detailed recipes for nutritious dinner options

1. Baked Salmon with Roasted Vegetables:

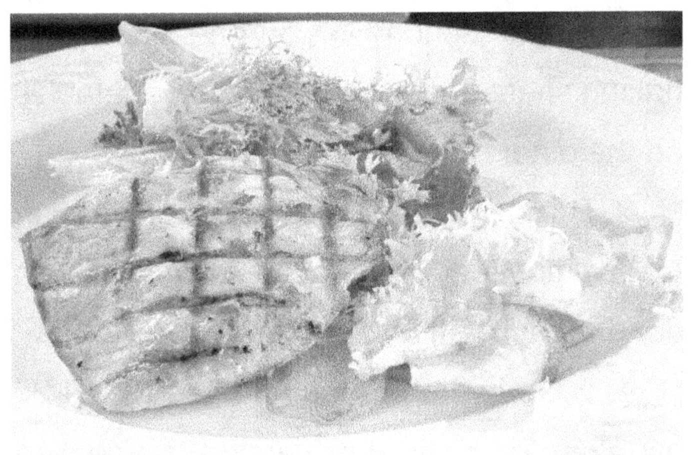

- Ingredients:

- 4 ounces salmon fillet

- 1 cup mixed vegetables (such as bell peppers, zucchini, cherry tomatoes, and broccoli florets)

- 1 tablespoon olive oil

- 1 teaspoon lemon juice

- 1 teaspoon dried herbs (such as dill, thyme, or rosemary)

- Salt and pepper to taste

- Instructions:

1. Preheat the oven to 400°F (200°C). Line a baking sheet with parchment paper.

2. Place salmon fillet on one side of the baking sheet and arrange mixed vegetables on the other side.

3. Drizzle olive oil and lemon juice over the salmon and vegetables. Sprinkle with dried herbs, salt, and pepper.

4. Bake in the preheated oven for 15-20 minutes, or until the salmon is cooked through and the vegetables are tender.

5. Serve hot with a side of whole grain rice or quinoa for a protein-rich and satisfying dinner option.

2. Turkey and Vegetable Stir-Fry:

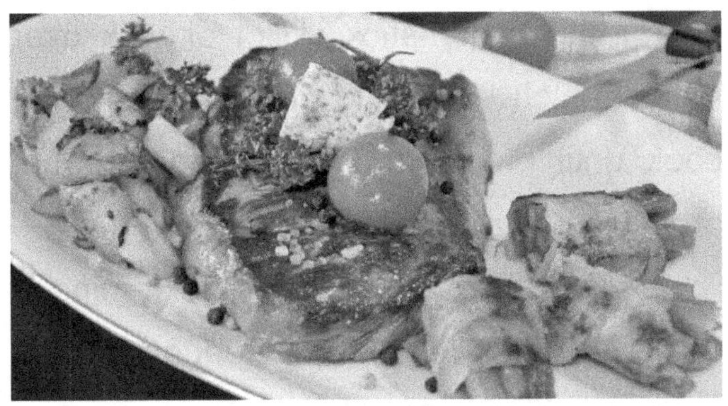

- Ingredients:

- 4 ounces lean ground turkey

- 2 cups mixed vegetables (such as bell peppers, snap peas, carrots, and broccoli florets)

- 2 cloves garlic, minced

- 1 tablespoon low-sodium soy sauce or tamari

- 1 teaspoon sesame oil

- 1/2 teaspoon ginger powder

- Cooked brown rice or quinoa for serving

- Optional toppings: chopped green onions, sesame seeds

- Instructions:

1. Heat a non-stick skillet or wok over medium-high heat. Add ground turkey and cook until browned and cooked through, breaking it apart with a spatula.

2. Add mixed vegetables and minced garlic to the skillet, stirring frequently, until the vegetables are tender-crisp.

3. In a small bowl, whisk together soy sauce or tamari, sesame oil, and ginger powder. Pour the sauce over the turkey and vegetables, stirring to coat evenly.

4. Cook for an additional 2-3 minutes, until the sauce has thickened slightly and everything is heated through.

5. Serve hot over cooked brown rice or quinoa, garnished with chopped green onions and sesame seeds if desired, for a flavorful and nutritious dinner option.

3. Veggie and Bean Chili:

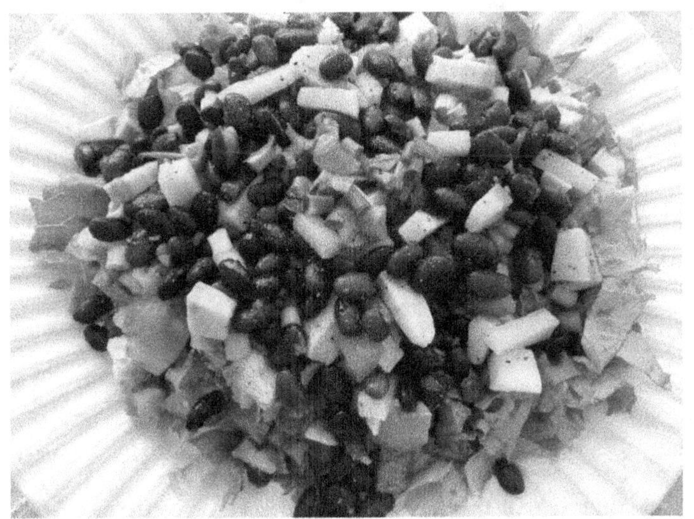

- Ingredients:

  - 1 tablespoon olive oil

  - 1 onion, chopped

  - 2 cloves garlic, minced

  - 1 bell pepper, chopped

  - 1 zucchini, chopped

  - 1 cup diced tomatoes (canned or fresh)

  - 1 cup low-sodium vegetable broth

  - 1 can (15 ounces) black beans, drained and rinsed

  - 1 can (15 ounces) kidney beans, drained and rinsed

- 1 tablespoon chili powder

- 1 teaspoon cumin

- Salt and pepper to taste

- Optional toppings: diced avocado, chopped cilantro, Greek yogurt or sour cream

- Instructions:

1. Heat olive oil in a large pot over medium heat. Add chopped onion and minced garlic, and sauté until softened and fragrant.

2. Add chopped bell pepper and zucchini to the pot, stirring occasionally, until vegetables are tender.

3. Stir in diced tomatoes, vegetable broth, black beans, kidney beans, chili powder, cumin, salt, and pepper. Bring to a simmer.

4. Reduce heat to low and simmer, uncovered, for 20-30 minutes, stirring occasionally, until flavors are well combined

and chili has thickened to your desired consistency.

5. Serve hot, garnished with diced avocado, chopped cilantro, and a dollop of Greek yogurt or sour cream if desired, for a hearty and satisfying dinner option.

4. Stuffed Bell Peppers with Quinoa and Turkey:

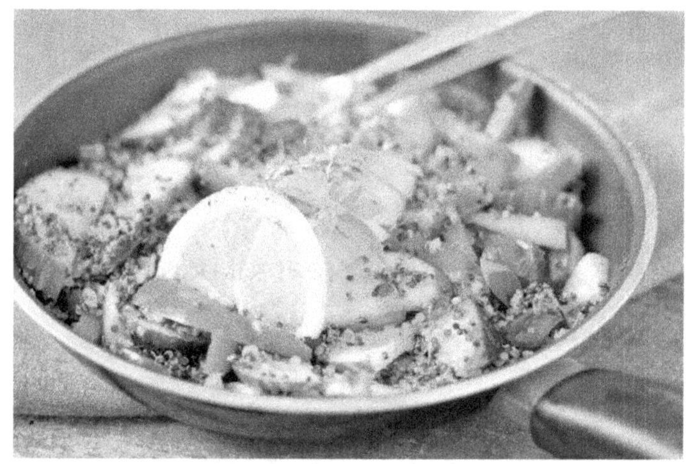

- Ingredients:

    - 4 large bell peppers, halved and seeds removed

    - 1 cup cooked quinoa

    - 8 ounces lean ground turkey

    - 1 cup diced tomatoes (canned or fresh)

    - 1/2 cup black beans, drained and rinsed

    - 1/2 cup corn kernels (fresh, canned, or frozen)

    - 1 teaspoon chili powder

    - 1/2 teaspoon cumin

    - Salt and pepper to taste

- Optional toppings: shredded cheese, chopped fresh cilantro

- Instructions:

1. Preheat the oven to 375°F (190°C). Arrange halved bell peppers in a baking dish, cut side up.

2. In a large skillet, cook ground turkey over medium heat until browned and cooked through. Drain excess fat if necessary.

3. Add cooked quinoa, diced tomatoes, black beans, corn kernels, chili powder, cumin, salt, and pepper to the skillet with the cooked turkey. Stir to combine.

4. Spoon the turkey and quinoa mixture into the halved bell peppers, filling each pepper evenly.

5. Cover the baking dish with foil and bake in the preheated oven for 30-35 minutes, or until the peppers are tender

.

6. Remove the foil and sprinkle shredded cheese over the stuffed peppers, if using. Return to the oven and bake for an additional 5 minutes, or until the cheese is melted and bubbly.

7. Serve hot, garnished with chopped fresh cilantro, for a wholesome and satisfying dinner option.

5. Eggplant and Chickpea Curry:

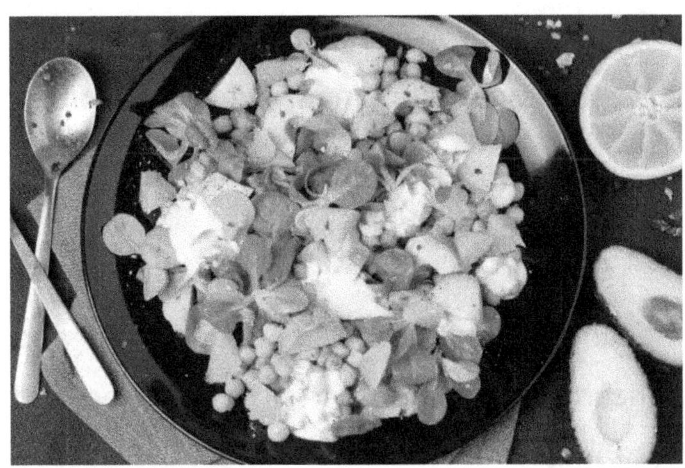

- Ingredients:

    - 1 tablespoon olive oil

    - 1 onion, chopped

    - 2 cloves garlic, minced

    - 1 eggplant, diced

    - 1 can (15 ounces) chickpeas, drained
and rinsed

    - 1 can (14 ounces) diced tomatoes

    - 1 cup low-sodium vegetable broth

    - 2 tablespoons curry powder

    - 1 teaspoon ground turmeric

    - 1 teaspoon ground cumin

    - Salt and pepper to taste

- Cooked brown rice or quinoa for serving

- Optional toppings: chopped fresh cilantro, Greek yogurt or coconut yogurt

- Instructions:

1. Heat olive oil in a large pot over medium heat. Add chopped onion and minced garlic, and sauté until softened and fragrant.

2. Add diced eggplant to the pot and cook until softened, stirring occasionally.

3. Stir in drained chickpeas, diced tomatoes, vegetable broth, curry powder, turmeric, cumin, salt, and pepper. Bring to a simmer.

4. Reduce heat to low and simmer, uncovered, for 20-25 minutes, stirring occasionally, until flavors are well combined and curry has thickened.

5. Serve hot over cooked brown rice or quinoa, garnished with chopped fresh cilantro and a dollop of Greek yogurt or

coconut yogurt if desired, for a flavorful and satisfying dinner option.

Adding these delicious and nutritious dinner recipes into your evening meal rotation can help you maintain a balanced and satisfying diet while following the DASH guidelines. By choosing whole, nutrient-dense ingredients and incorporating a variety of flavors and textures, you can enjoy nourishing meals that support your health and well-being. Experiment with different recipes and adapt them to suit your taste preferences and dietary needs for a truly enjoyable dinner experience.

Chapter Four: Snacks and Desserts for Seniors on the DASH Diet

Healthy Snack Ideas

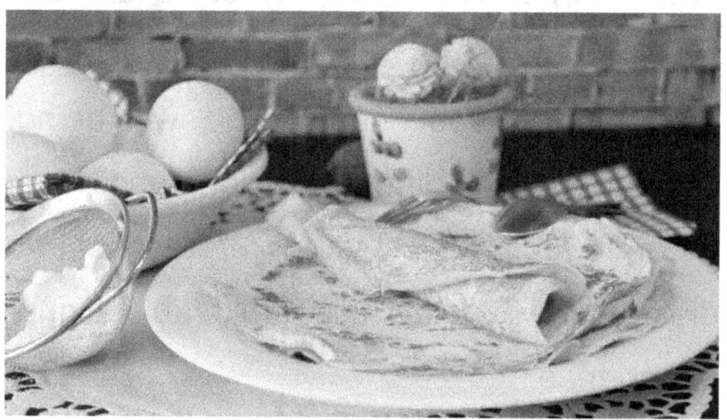

Snacking can be an essential part of a healthy diet, providing an opportunity to curb hunger between meals, boost energy levels, and satisfy cravings. When following the Dietary Approaches to Stop Hypertension

(DASH) diet, it's important to choose snacks that are not only delicious but also nutrient-dense and aligned with the principles of the DASH diet. Below are detailed ideas for healthy snacks that are perfect for DASH diet followers:

1. Fresh Fruit with Nut Butter:

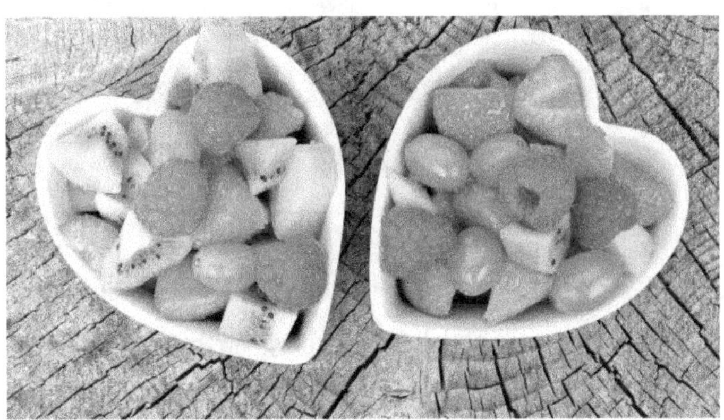

- Pairing fresh fruits like apple slices, banana, or pear with a tablespoon of almond butter, peanut butter, or cashew butter provides a satisfying combination of natural sweetness, fiber, and healthy fats. Choose nut butters without added sugars or hydrogenated oils for the healthiest option.

2. Greek Yogurt with Berries:

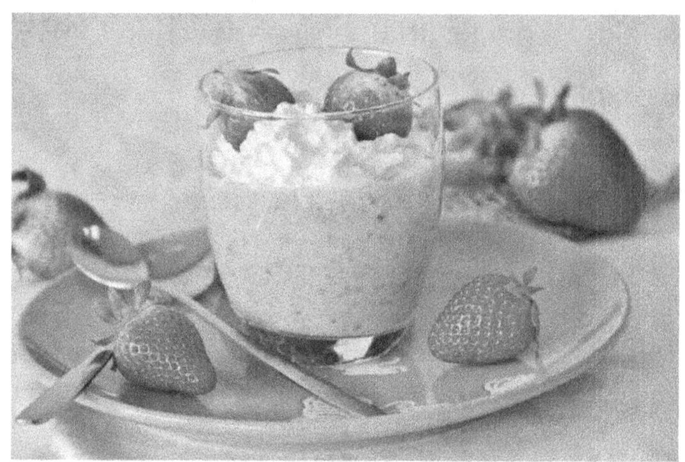

- Enjoy a serving of plain Greek yogurt topped with a handful of fresh berries such as strawberries, blueberries, or raspberries. Greek yogurt is high in protein and probiotics, while berries are packed with antioxidants and fiber, making this snack both nutritious and satisfying.

3. Veggie Sticks with Hummus:

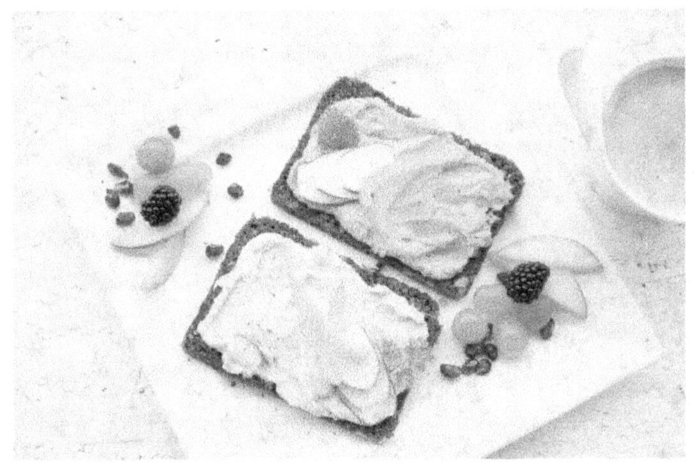

- Cut up crunchy vegetables like carrot sticks, cucumber slices, bell pepper strips, and celery sticks, and serve with a side of homemade or store-bought hummus. Vegetables are rich in vitamins, minerals, and fiber, while hummus provides protein and healthy fats, making this a balanced and filling snack option.

4. Whole Grain Crackers with Cottage Cheese:

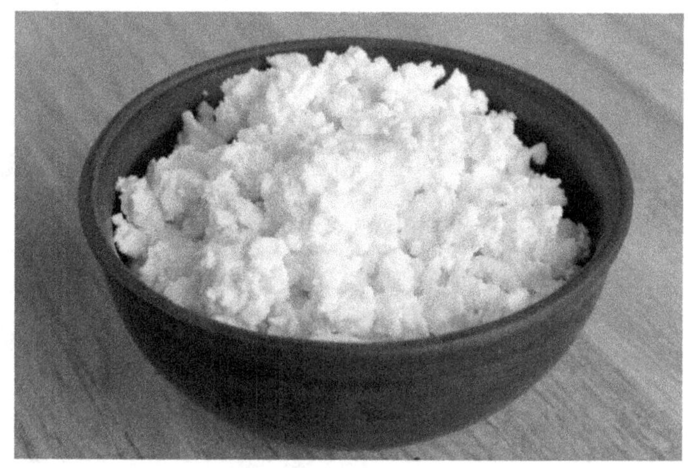

- Enjoy a serving of whole grain crackers topped with a dollop of low-fat cottage cheese and a sprinkle of herbs or spices. Whole grain crackers provide fiber and complex carbohydrates, while cottage cheese offers protein and calcium, making this snack both satisfying and nutritious.

5. Trail Mix with Nuts and Seeds:

- Mix together a handful of unsalted nuts (such as almonds, walnuts, or pistachios) with seeds (such as pumpkin seeds or sunflower seeds) and a small serving of dried fruit (such as raisins, apricots, or cranberries) to create a homemade trail mix. This snack provides a combination of protein, healthy fats, and carbohydrates, making it an ideal option for sustained energy.

6. Cottage Cheese with Pineapple:

- Combine a serving of low-fat cottage cheese with chunks of fresh pineapple for a sweet and creamy snack. Cottage cheese is rich in protein and calcium, while pineapple provides natural sweetness and vitamin C, making this a refreshing and satisfying option.

7. Hard-Boiled Eggs:

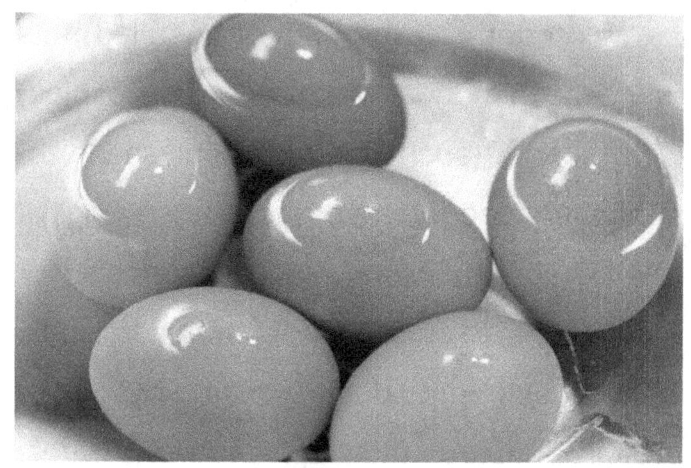

- Hard-boiled eggs are a convenient and portable snack that provides protein, vitamins, and minerals. Enjoy one or two hard-boiled eggs seasoned with a sprinkle of salt and pepper for a quick and satisfying snack option.

8. Whole Grain Toast with Avocado:

- Toast a slice of whole grain bread and top it with mashed avocado for a nutrient-dense and satisfying snack. Avocado is rich in heart-healthy fats, while whole grain bread provides fiber and complex carbohydrates, making this a filling and delicious option.

9. Edamame:

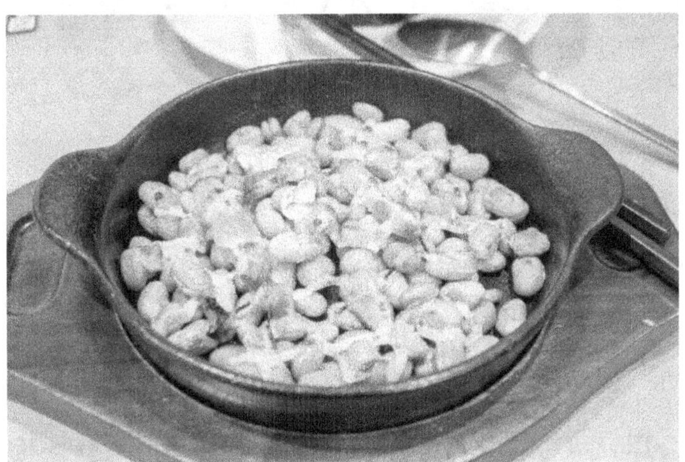

- Enjoy a serving of steamed edamame (young soybeans) sprinkled with a pinch of sea salt for a protein-rich and satisfying snack. Edamame is a good source of plant-based protein, fiber, and essential nutrients, making it an excellent option for DASH diet followers.

10. Cucumber Slices with Tzatziki:

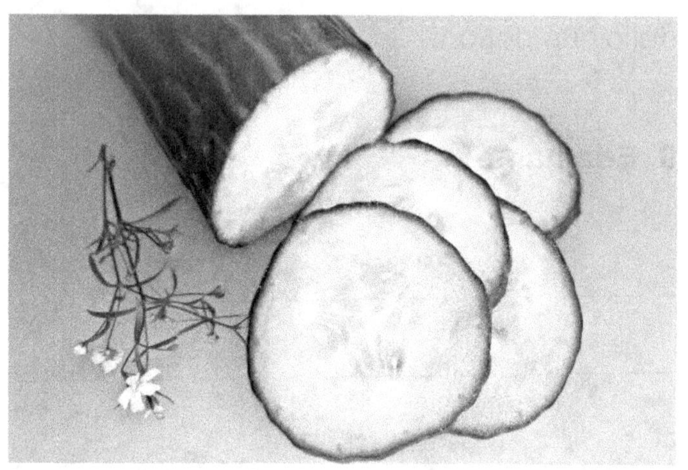

- Slice a cucumber and serve it with a side of tzatziki sauce for a refreshing and satisfying snack. Tzatziki sauce is made from Greek yogurt, cucumber, garlic, and herbs, providing protein, probiotics, and flavor, while cucumber adds hydration and crunch.

Including these healthy snack ideas into your daily routine can help you stay satisfied and energized while following the DASH diet. By choosing nutrient-dense options that are rich in protein, fiber, and healthy fats, you can support your overall health and well-being while satisfying your cravings between meals. Experiment with different combinations and flavors to find the snacks that work best for you, and enjoy the benefits of a balanced and nutritious diet.

Dessert Recipes with DASH Diet Twist

While following the Dietary Approaches to Stop Hypertension (DASH) diet, you don't have to sacrifice enjoying delicious desserts. By incorporating nutrient-dense ingredients and making mindful choices, you can create sweet treats that satisfy your cravings while still aligning with the principles of the DASH diet. Below are detailed dessert recipes with a DASH diet twist:

1. Berry Chia Seed Pudding:

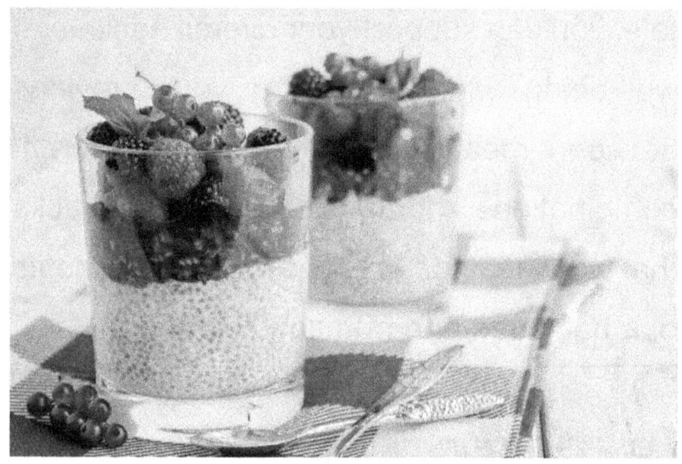

- Ingredients:

  - 1/4 cup chia seeds

  - 1 cup unsweetened almond milk or low-fat milk

  - 1 tablespoon honey or maple syrup

  - 1/2 teaspoon vanilla extract

  - 1 cup mixed berries (such as strawberries, blueberries, and raspberries)

- Instructions:

  1. In a mixing bowl, combine chia seeds, almond milk, honey or maple syrup, and vanilla extract. Stir well to combine.

2. Let the mixture sit for 5 minutes, then stir again to prevent clumping. Repeat this process a few times until the chia seeds have absorbed the liquid and the mixture has thickened to a pudding-like consistency.

3. In serving glasses or bowls, layer the chia seed pudding with mixed berries.

4. Refrigerate for at least 2 hours or overnight to allow the flavors to meld and the pudding to set.

5. Serve chilled as a refreshing and nutritious dessert option.

2. Banana Oat Cookies:

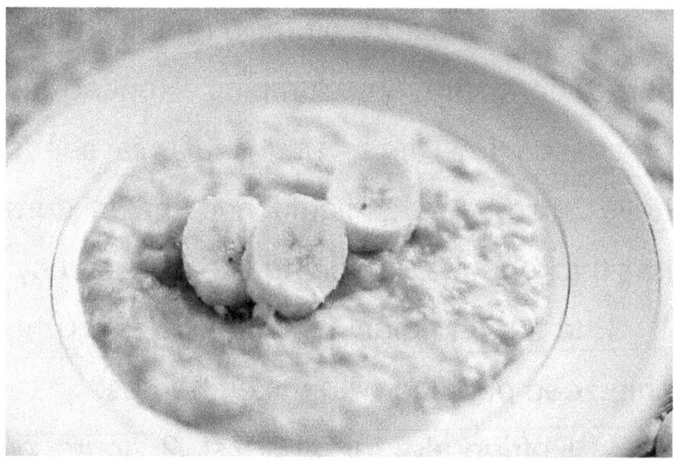

- Ingredients:

    - 2 ripe bananas, mashed

    - 1 cup rolled oats

    - 1/4 cup chopped nuts (such as almonds
or walnuts)

    - 1/4 cup raisins or dried cranberries

    - 1 teaspoon cinnamon

    - 1/2 teaspoon vanilla extract

- Instructions:

    1. Preheat the oven to 350°F (175°C).
Line a baking sheet with parchment paper.

    2. In a mixing bowl, combine mashed
bananas, rolled oats, chopped nuts, raisins

or dried cranberries, cinnamon, and vanilla extract. Stir until well combined.

3. Drop spoonfuls of the cookie dough onto the prepared baking sheet, spacing them apart.

4. Flatten each cookie with the back of a spoon or fork to shape them.

5. Bake in the preheated oven for 12-15 minutes, or until the cookies are golden brown and set.

6. Allow the cookies to cool on the baking sheet for a few minutes before transferring them to a wire rack to cool completely.

7. Enjoy these wholesome cookies as a guilt-free dessert or snack option.

3. Dark Chocolate-Dipped Strawberries:

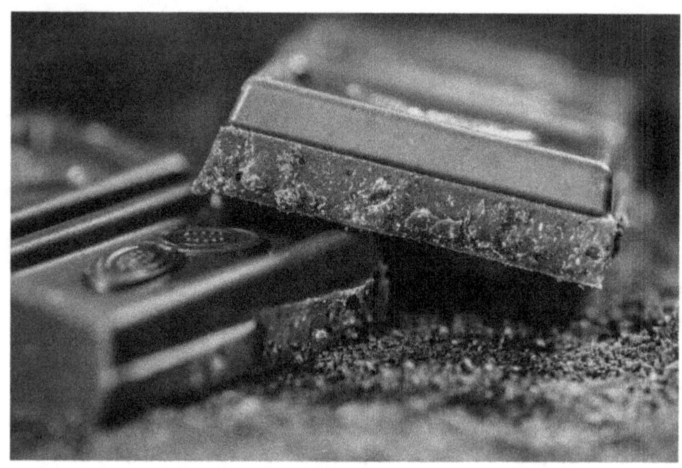

- Ingredients:

  - 1 cup fresh strawberries, washed and dried

  - 1/4 cup dark chocolate chips

  - 1 teaspoon coconut oil

- Instructions:

  1. Line a baking sheet with parchment paper.

  2. In a microwave-safe bowl, combine dark chocolate chips and coconut oil. Microwave in 30-second intervals, stirring in between, until the chocolate is melted and smooth.

3. Holding each strawberry by the stem, dip it into the melted chocolate, allowing any excess chocolate to drip off.

4. Place the chocolate-dipped strawberries on the prepared baking sheet.

5. Refrigerate for 10-15 minutes, or until the chocolate is set.

6. Enjoy these decadent treats as a delicious and antioxidant-rich dessert option.

4. Greek Yogurt Parfait with Granola and Fruit:

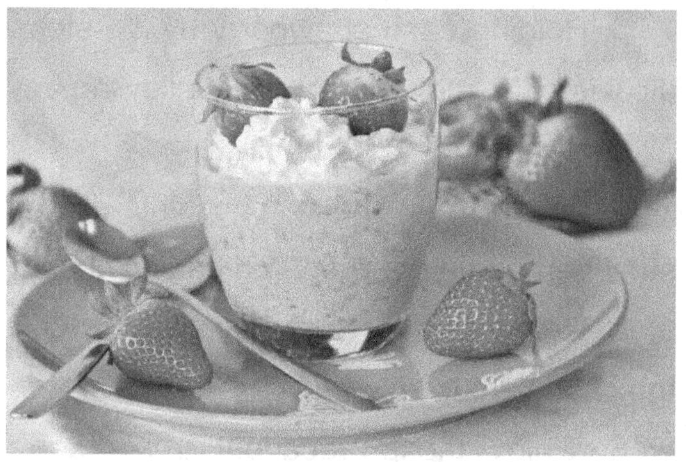

- Ingredients:

 - 1/2 cup plain Greek yogurt

 - 1/4 cup granola (choose a low-sugar, whole grain variety)

 - 1/4 cup mixed fresh fruit (such as berries, sliced banana, or diced mango)

 - 1 tablespoon honey or maple syrup (optional)

- Instructions:

1. In a serving glass or bowl, layer Greek yogurt, granola, and mixed fresh fruit.

2. Drizzle with honey or maple syrup, if desired, for added sweetness.

3. Repeat the layers until the glass or bowl is filled to your liking.

4. Serve immediately as a satisfying and protein-rich dessert option.

5. Baked Apples with Cinnamon and Nuts:

- Ingredients:

  - 2 apples, cored and halved

  - 1 tablespoon chopped nuts (such as pecans or almonds)

  - 1 teaspoon cinnamon

  - 1 teaspoon honey or maple syrup

- Instructions:

1. Preheat the oven to 375°F (190°C). Line a baking dish with parchment paper.

2. Place the apple halves in the prepared baking dish, cut side up.

3. In a small bowl, combine chopped nuts, cinnamon, and honey or maple syrup. Mix well.

4. Spoon the nut mixture evenly into the cavities of the apple halves.

5. Bake in the preheated oven for 20-25 minutes, or until the apples are tender and golden brown.

6. Serve hot as a comforting and naturally sweet dessert option.

These delightful dessert recipes with a DASH diet twist allow you to indulge in sweet treats while still prioritizing your health and well-being. By using wholesome ingredients and making mindful choices, you can satisfy your cravings without compromising your dietary goals. Experiment with these recipes and get creative with variations to discover your favorite guilt-free desserts. Enjoy the sweet side of life while staying true to the principles of the DASH diet.

Staying hydrated and nourished is essential for seniors to maintain optimal health and well-being. Incorporating nutrient-rich beverages and smoothies into their diet can provide hydration, essential vitamins, minerals, and antioxidants while following the Dietary Approaches to Stop Hypertension (DASH) diet principles. Below are detailed ideas for beverages and smoothies tailored to seniors on the DASH diet:

1. Green Power Smoothie:

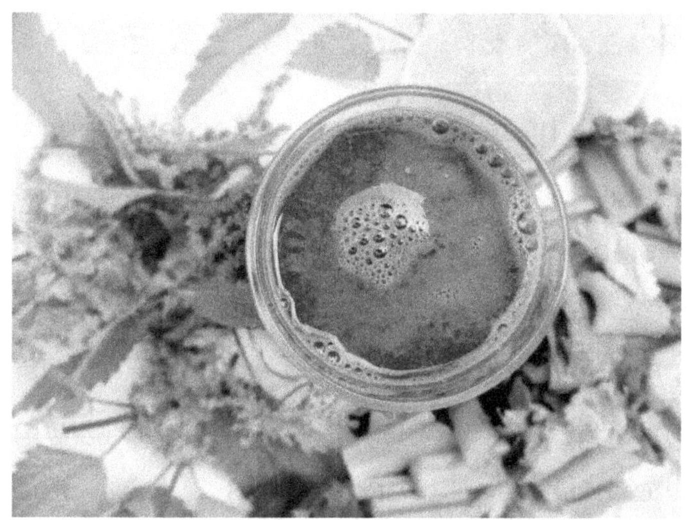

- Ingredients:

    - 1 cup spinach or kale, fresh or frozen

    - 1/2 cup cucumber, chopped

    - 1/2 banana, frozen

    - 1/2 cup pineapple chunks, frozen

    - 1/2 cup unsweetened almond milk or low-fat milk

    - 1/2 cup plain Greek yogurt

    - 1 tablespoon chia seeds or ground flaxseeds

    - Optional: honey or maple syrup for sweetness

- Instructions:

1. Combine all ingredients in a blender.

2. Blend until smooth and creamy.

3. Pour into a glass and enjoy immediately as a refreshing and nutrient-packed smoothie option.

2. Berry Blast Smoothie:

- Ingredients:

- 1/2 cup mixed berries (such as strawberries, blueberries, and raspberries), fresh or frozen

- 1/2 banana, frozen

- 1/2 cup spinach or kale

- 1/2 cup plain Greek yogurt

- 1/2 cup unsweetened almond milk or low-fat milk

- 1 tablespoon almond butter or peanut butter

- Optional: honey or maple syrup for sweetness

- Instructions:

1. Place all ingredients in a blender.

2. Blend until smooth and creamy.

3. Pour into a glass and serve immediately as a delicious and antioxidant-rich smoothie option.

3. Golden Turmeric Latte:

- Ingredients:

- 1 cup unsweetened almond milk or low-fat milk

- 1/2 teaspoon ground turmeric

- 1/4 teaspoon ground cinnamon

- 1/4 teaspoon ground ginger

- 1 teaspoon honey or maple syrup

- Optional: a pinch of black pepper (to enhance turmeric absorption)

- Instructions:

1. In a small saucepan, heat almond milk or low-fat milk over medium heat until warm but not boiling.

2. Whisk in ground turmeric, cinnamon, ginger, and honey or maple syrup until well combined.

3. Continue to heat for a few minutes, stirring occasionally, until the mixture is hot and frothy.

4. Pour the golden turmeric latte into a mug and sprinkle with a pinch of black pepper, if desired.

5. Serve immediately as a comforting and anti-inflammatory beverage option.

4. Tropical Coconut Water Smoothie:

- Ingredients:

    - 1/2 cup coconut water

    - 1/2 cup pineapple chunks, fresh or frozen

    - 1/2 banana, frozen

    - 1/4 cup mango chunks, fresh or frozen

    - 1/2 cup plain Greek yogurt

- 1 tablespoon shredded coconut (unsweetened)

- Optional: a squeeze of lime juice for brightness

- Instructions:

1. Combine all ingredients in a blender.

2. Blend until smooth and creamy.

3. Pour into a glass and garnish with additional shredded coconut or a slice of lime, if desired.

4. Serve immediately as a tropical and hydrating smoothie option.

5. Veggie Boost Juice:

- Ingredients:

    - 1 large carrot, peeled and chopped

    - 1/2 cucumber, chopped

    - 1 stalk celery, chopped

    - 1/2 apple, cored and chopped

    - 1/2 lemon, juiced

    - 1/2-inch piece of ginger, peeled

- 1 cup water or coconut water

- Optional: a handful of spinach or kale for added greens

- Instructions:

1. Place all ingredients in a juicer or high-speed blender.

2. Blend or juice until smooth.

3. Strain the mixture through a fine-mesh sieve to remove any pulp, if desired.

4. Pour into a glass and serve immediately as a refreshing and nutrient-packed juice option.

6. Minty Green Tea Cooler:

- Ingredients:

  - 1 cup brewed green tea, chilled

  - 1/4 cup fresh mint leaves

  - 1/2 lemon, juiced

  - 1 teaspoon honey or maple syrup

  - Ice cubes

- Instructions:

1. In a blender, combine chilled green tea, fresh mint leaves, lemon juice, and honey or maple syrup.

2. Blend until the mint is finely chopped and the mixture is well combined.

3. Fill a glass with ice cubes and pour the minty green tea mixture over the ice.

4. Garnish with a sprig of fresh mint and a slice of lemon, if desired.

5. Serve immediately as a refreshing and antioxidant-rich beverage option.

Incorporating these flavorful beverages and nutrient-packed smoothies into the diet of seniors following the DASH guidelines can provide hydration, essential nutrients, and a delicious way to stay healthy. By choosing wholesome ingredients and experimenting with different flavors and combinations, seniors can enjoy refreshing beverages and smoothies that support their overall well-being while adhering to the principles of the DASH diet. Stay hydrated, nourished, and energized with these delightful options tailored to seniors' dietary needs.

Chapter Five: Special Considerations for Seniors on the DASH Diet

Managing Chronic Conditions with the DASH Diet

Chronic conditions such as hypertension, heart disease, diabetes, and obesity are prevalent among individuals of all ages, particularly seniors. However, adopting a healthy lifestyle, including dietary modifications, can play a significant role in managing these conditions and improving overall health and well-being. The Dietary Approaches to Stop Hypertension (DASH) diet has emerged as an effective dietary approach for managing chronic conditions due to its focus on nutrient-rich foods and its ability to promote heart health, lower blood pressure, and support weight management. Below is a detailed overview of how the DASH diet can help manage chronic conditions:

1. Lowering Blood Pressure:

- High blood pressure, or hypertension, is a common chronic condition that increases the risk of heart disease, stroke, and other health complications. The DASH diet emphasizes consuming foods rich in potassium, calcium, magnesium, and fiber while limiting sodium intake, which has been shown to help lower blood pressure levels. By prioritizing fruits, vegetables, whole grains, lean proteins, and low-fat dairy products, individuals following the DASH diet can effectively manage hypertension and reduce their risk of cardiovascular disease.

2. Supporting Heart Health:

- Heart disease is a leading cause of morbidity and mortality worldwide, especially among seniors. The DASH diet promotes heart health by encouraging the consumption of nutrient-dense foods that are low in saturated fats, cholesterol, and refined sugars. By focusing on a diet rich in fruits, vegetables, whole grains, lean proteins, and healthy fats, individuals can reduce their risk of developing heart disease and improve their overall cardiovascular health.

3. Managing Diabetes:

- Diabetes is a chronic condition characterized by elevated blood sugar levels, which can lead to serious complications such as heart disease, kidney disease, and nerve damage. The DASH diet, with its emphasis on whole, unprocessed foods and balanced macronutrient intake, can be beneficial for individuals with diabetes. By regulating blood sugar levels and promoting weight management, the DASH diet can help individuals with diabetes better control their condition and reduce the risk of complications.

4. Promoting Weight Management:

- Obesity is a significant risk factor for many chronic conditions, including heart disease, diabetes, and hypertension. The DASH diet can support weight management efforts by encouraging the consumption of nutrient-dense foods that are low in calories and high in fiber. By focusing on portion control, limiting the intake of high-calorie, processed foods, and incorporating regular physical activity, individuals following the DASH diet can achieve and maintain a healthy weight, reducing the risk of obesity-related complications.

5. Improving Overall Nutrition:

   - Many chronic conditions are influenced by dietary factors, making nutrition a critical component of disease management and prevention. The DASH diet provides a well-rounded approach to nutrition by promoting the consumption of a variety of nutrient-rich foods from all food groups. By emphasizing whole, minimally processed foods and reducing the intake of unhealthy fats, sugars, and sodium, individuals can improve their overall nutritional status and support their body's natural healing and disease-fighting abilities.

6. Enhancing Quality of Life:

- Managing chronic conditions can significantly impact an individual's quality of life, affecting their physical health, emotional well-being, and daily functioning. By adopting a health-promoting lifestyle that includes following the DASH diet, individuals can experience improvements in energy levels, mood, and overall vitality. By nourishing their bodies with wholesome foods and engaging in regular physical activity, individuals can better manage their chronic conditions and enjoy a higher quality of life as they age.

The DASH diet offers a holistic approach to managing chronic conditions by emphasizing nutrient-rich foods, portion control, and lifestyle modifications. By following the principles of the DASH diet, individuals can effectively lower blood pressure, support heart health, manage diabetes, promote weight management, improve overall nutrition, and enhance their quality of life. With its focus on balanced eating patterns and sustainable lifestyle changes, the DASH diet serves as a valuable tool for individuals looking to take control of their health and well-being, particularly those managing chronic conditions in their senior years.

DASH Diet and Medication Interactions for Seniors

For seniors managing chronic conditions such as hypertension, heart disease, and diabetes, medication plays a crucial role in controlling symptoms and preventing complications. However, dietary choices can also impact the effectiveness and safety of medications, including those commonly prescribed to seniors. The Dietary Approaches to Stop Hypertension (DASH) diet, known for its focus on nutrient-rich foods and its potential to improve health outcomes, may interact with certain medications, necessitating careful consideration and monitoring. Below is a detailed exploration of DASH diet and medication interactions for seniors:

1. Blood Pressure Medications:

   - Seniors with hypertension often take medications such as angiotensin-converting enzyme (ACE) inhibitors, angiotensin II receptor blockers (ARBs), beta-blockers, diuretics, and calcium channel blockers to lower blood pressure. The DASH diet, which emphasizes fruits, vegetables, whole grains, lean proteins, and low-fat dairy products while limiting sodium intake, can complement these medications by further lowering blood pressure. However, sudden and significant changes in dietary sodium intake may affect the effectiveness of certain blood pressure medications, particularly diuretics. Seniors should work closely with their healthcare provider to monitor blood pressure levels and adjust medication dosages as needed when adopting the DASH diet.

2. Diabetes Medications:

- Seniors with diabetes may take medications such as insulin, sulfonylureas, metformin, and dipeptidyl peptidase-4 (DPP-4) inhibitors to regulate blood sugar levels. The DASH diet, with its emphasis on whole, unprocessed foods and balanced macronutrient intake, can support blood sugar management and improve insulin sensitivity. However, seniors taking diabetes medications should be aware that certain

DASH diet components, such as fruits and whole grains, may impact blood sugar levels. Regular monitoring of blood glucose levels and close communication with healthcare providers are essential to ensure the safe and effective management of diabetes while following the DASH diet.

3. Cholesterol-Lowering Medications:

- Seniors with high cholesterol levels may take medications such as statins, bile acid sequestrants, and PCSK9 inhibitors to lower cholesterol levels and reduce the risk of heart disease. The DASH diet, which promotes heart-healthy foods such as fruits, vegetables, whole grains, and lean proteins, can complement cholesterol-lowering medications by further improving lipid profiles and cardiovascular health. However, seniors should be cautious when combining certain cholesterol-lowering medications with grapefruit, as it contains compounds that can interfere with the metabolism of these drugs. Seniors should consult with their healthcare provider or pharmacist to determine if any dietary restrictions apply to their specific medication regimen.

4. Anticoagulant Medications:

- Seniors taking anticoagulant medications such as warfarin (Coumadin) to prevent blood clots should be mindful of their vitamin K intake when following the DASH diet. Vitamin K, found in leafy green vegetables such as spinach, kale, and broccoli, can interfere with the anticoagulant effects of warfarin. While these vitamin K-rich foods are central to the DASH diet's focus on plant-based nutrition, seniors on warfarin may need to monitor their intake of these foods and maintain consistent levels to avoid fluctuations in medication effectiveness. Healthcare providers can provide guidance on incorporating vitamin K-rich foods into the diet while managing anticoagulant therapy.

5. NSAIDs and Blood Pressure:

- Nonsteroidal anti-inflammatory drugs (NSAIDs) such as ibuprofen and naproxen are commonly used by seniors to relieve pain and inflammation. However, prolonged use of NSAIDs may lead to fluid retention and increased blood pressure, which can counteract the benefits of the DASH diet in managing hypertension. Seniors should use NSAIDs cautiously and under the guidance of a healthcare provider, particularly if they are following the DASH diet to lower blood pressure. Alternatives to NSAIDs, such as acetaminophen, may be recommended for pain management in seniors with hypertension or other cardiovascular risk factors.

While the DASH diet offers numerous health benefits for seniors, including improved blood pressure control, heart health, and overall well-being, it is essential to consider potential interactions with medications commonly used by this population. Seniors should work closely with their healthcare providers to monitor medication effectiveness, adjust dosages as needed, and make informed dietary choices that support their health goals while minimizing the risk of adverse interactions. By staying informed and proactive, seniors can safely integrate the DASH diet into their medication regimen and optimize their health outcomes for years to come.

Staying Active and Fit: Exercise Tips for Seniors

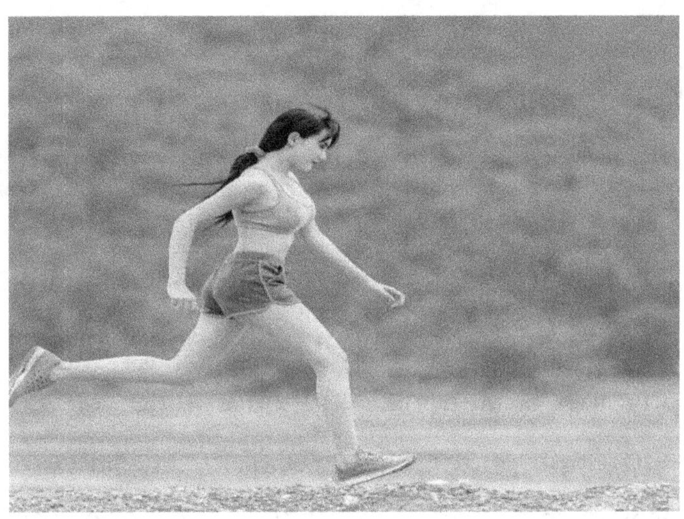

Physical activity plays a crucial role in maintaining health and well-being, especially for seniors who are following the Dietary Approaches to Stop Hypertension (DASH) diet. Regular exercise not only complements the benefits of the DASH diet in managing chronic conditions such as hypertension, heart disease, and diabetes but also supports overall physical function, mobility, and quality of life. Below are detailed exercise tips tailored to seniors following the DASH diet:

1. Consult with Your Healthcare Provider:

- Before starting any exercise program, seniors should consult with their healthcare provider to assess their overall health status, identify any underlying medical conditions or physical limitations, and determine a safe and appropriate exercise plan. Healthcare providers can provide personalized recommendations based on individual health needs and goals, ensuring that exercise complements the DASH diet in promoting optimal health.

2. Focus on Cardiovascular Exercise:

- Cardiovascular exercise, also known as aerobic exercise, is essential for seniors to improve heart health, boost endurance, and manage weight. Engaging in activities such as brisk walking, cycling, swimming, dancing, or using cardio machines at the gym can help seniors meet the recommended guidelines for aerobic exercise, which include at least 150 minutes of moderate-intensity exercise or 75 minutes of vigorous-intensity exercise per week. Incorporating cardiovascular exercise into your routine complements the DASH diet's focus on heart-healthy eating patterns, promoting overall cardiovascular health and well-being.

3. Include Strength Training:

- Strength training, or resistance exercise, is crucial for seniors to maintain muscle mass, strength, and bone density, which tend to decline with age. Incorporating exercises such as bodyweight exercises, resistance band exercises, or weightlifting can help seniors build and maintain muscle strength, improve balance, and reduce the risk of falls and fractures. Strength training also complements the DASH diet by supporting weight management and improving overall physical function and mobility.

4. Prioritize Flexibility and Balance Exercises:

- Flexibility and balance exercises are essential for seniors to maintain joint mobility, flexibility, and stability, reducing the risk of falls and injuries. Activities such as yoga, tai chi, Pilates, or simple stretching exercises can help seniors improve flexibility, enhance balance and coordination, and promote relaxation and stress reduction. Incorporating flexibility and balance exercises into your routine enhances overall physical function and complements the DASH diet's focus on holistic health and well-being.

5. Start Slow and Progress Gradually:

- Seniors should start any new exercise program slowly and progress gradually to prevent injury and avoid overexertion. Begin with low-impact activities and light resistance exercises, gradually increasing intensity, duration, and frequency as your fitness level improves. Listening to your body, paying attention to any signs of discomfort or fatigue, and adjusting your exercise routine accordingly is essential for long-term success. By starting slow and progressing gradually, seniors can build confidence, improve fitness, and enjoy the benefits of regular exercise while following the DASH diet.

6. Stay Hydrated and Fuel Your Body Properly:

- Proper hydration and nutrition are essential for supporting exercise performance, recovery, and overall health, especially for seniors following the DASH diet. Drink plenty of water before, during, and after exercise to stay hydrated and replace fluids lost through sweat. Additionally, fuel your body with nutrient-dense foods that provide energy, such as fruits, vegetables, whole grains, lean proteins, and healthy fats. By staying hydrated and properly fueled, seniors can optimize exercise performance, support recovery, and enhance the benefits of the DASH diet for overall health and well-being.

7. Listen to Your Body and Rest as Needed:

- It's essential for seniors to listen to their bodies and rest as needed during exercise. Pay attention to any signs of fatigue, dizziness, or discomfort, and take breaks or modify exercises accordingly. Rest and recovery are crucial for preventing overuse injuries and allowing the body to adapt and repair itself after exercise. By listening to your body and honoring your limits, you can maintain a safe and sustainable exercise routine that complements the DASH diet and supports long-term health and well-being.

Staying active and fit is essential for seniors to maintain health, mobility, and independence, especially when following the DASH diet to manage chronic conditions. By incorporating cardiovascular exercise, strength training, flexibility and balance exercises, and restorative activities into their routine, seniors can optimize their physical function, improve overall health, and enhance the benefits of the DASH diet. By consulting with healthcare providers, starting slow, and listening to their bodies, seniors can create a safe and effective exercise plan that supports their unique health needs and goals for active aging.

Conclusion

As we reach the end, it's essential to reflect on the significance of nourishing our bodies with wholesome, nutrient-rich foods and adopting healthy lifestyle habits. Throughout this cookbook, we've explored the principles of the DASH diet and how they can benefit seniors by promoting heart health, managing chronic conditions, and supporting overall well-being. From delicious recipes to practical tips for meal planning, preparation, and incorporating physical activity, we've provided a comprehensive guide to help seniors make positive changes to their dietary habits and lifestyle.

Reflecting on the DASH Diet Journey:

- The journey through the DASH diet cookbook has been one of discovery, empowerment, and transformation. By embracing the principles of the DASH diet – focusing on fruits, vegetables, whole grains, lean proteins, and healthy fats while limiting sodium, refined sugars, and unhealthy fats – seniors have learned how to nourish their bodies with delicious, nutrient-dense foods that promote optimal health and vitality.

Celebrating Health and Well-Being:

- As seniors embrace the DASH diet and incorporate its principles into their daily lives, they celebrate not only improved physical health but also enhanced emotional well-being and quality of life. By fueling their bodies with wholesome foods and staying active, seniors can enjoy increased energy levels, improved mood, better sleep, and a greater sense of vitality and purpose.

Empowering Seniors to Take Charge of Their Health:

- This cookbook empowers seniors to take charge of their health and make informed choices that support their unique dietary needs and goals. By providing a variety of delicious and nutritious recipes, along with practical tips for meal planning, preparation, and physical activity, seniors have the tools they need to create a healthy and fulfilling lifestyle that aligns with the principles of the DASH diet.

Looking Ahead:

- As seniors continue their journey with the DASH diet, they can look forward to continued improvements in their health and well-being. By staying committed to a balanced and nutritious diet, incorporating regular physical activity, and maintaining a positive outlook on life, seniors can thrive in their golden years and enjoy a vibrant and active lifestyle for years to come.

Gratitude and Appreciation:

- Finally, we express our gratitude and appreciation to all seniors who have embarked on this journey with us. Your dedication to embracing the DASH diet and prioritizing your health and wellness is truly inspiring. We hope that the recipes, tips, and information provided in this cookbook have enriched your life and empowered you to live your best life possible.